DIAGNOSTIC PICTURE TESTS IN

PAEDIATRIC DENTISTRY

W. P. Rock
DDS, FDS, D.Orth.RCS
Senior Lecturer and Honorary Consultant

Margaret C. Grundy
DDS, FDS.RCS
Senior Lecturer

Linda Shaw
BDS, PhD, FDS.RCS
Senior Lecturer and Honorary Consultant

Department of Children's Dentistry and Orthodontics
University of Birmingham, England

Wolfe Medical Publications Ltd

Titles in this series, published or being developed, include:
Diagnostic Picture Tests in Paediatrics
Picture Tests in Human Anatomy
Diagnostic Picture Tests in Oral Medicine
Diagnostic Picture Tests in Orthopaedics
Diagnostic Picture Tests in Infectious Diseases
Diagnostic Picture Tests in Dermatology
Diagnostic Picture Tests in Ophthalmology
Diagnostic Picture Tests in Rheumatology
Diagnostic Picture Tests in Obstetrics/Gynaecology
Diagnostic Picture Tests in Clinical Neurology
Diagnostic Picture Tests in Injury in Sport
Diagnostic Picture Tests in General Surgery
Diagnostic Picture Tests in General Medicine
Diagnostic Picture Tests in Paediatric Dentistry
Diagnostic Picture Tests in Dentistry
Picture Tests in Embryology

Copyright © W. Rock, M. Grundy & L. Shaw, 1988
First published 1988 by Wolfe Medical Publications Ltd
Printed by BPCC Hazell Books, Aylesbury, England
ISBN 0 7234 0984 6
Reprinted 1991

For a full list of Wolfe Medical Atlases, plus
forthcoming titles and details of our surgical,
dental and veterinary Atlases, please write to
Wolfe Medical Publications Limited,
2-16 Torrington Place, London WC1E 7LT.

000192

WM 480 Roc
14/5/92

Preface

This book covers a wide range of conditions likely· to be seen by those concerned with child patients. They include developmental anomalies of tooth formation, soft tissue lesions and systemic conditions related to dentistry. Some more rarely encountered craniofacial abnormalities are also shown.

In common with the other specialities in this series, the illustrations are presented in random order rather than by subject to achieve a more effective testing procedure. Maximum benefit will be derived if full answers are written before reference is made to the back of the book.

Acknowledgements

Most of the illustrations are of patients seen by the authors. Additional material has been generously provided by Professor T D Foster, Mr M J C Wake and the West Midland Craniofacial Unit, Mr H D Glenwright and Dr M K Basu. Picture 81 is used with the permission of the British Journal of Hospital Medicine.

We would like to thank Mr M Sharland and Mr C Rice of the Photographic Unit and members of the Department of Clinical Illustration, University of Birmingham for kind and expert help. We are most grateful to Mrs Michelle Bailey who prepared the manuscript so efficiently.

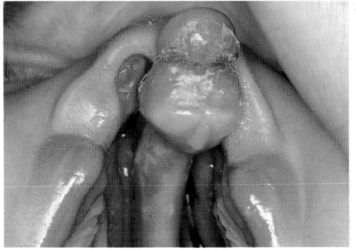

1 An 11-year-old child fell three weeks ago.
(a) What has produced this appearance?
(b) What treatment is necessary?

2 This baby has a bilateral cleft of lip and palate.
(a) When would the defects normally be repaired?
(b) What dental problems may present later?

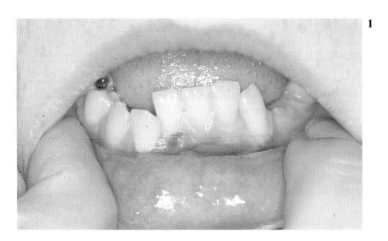

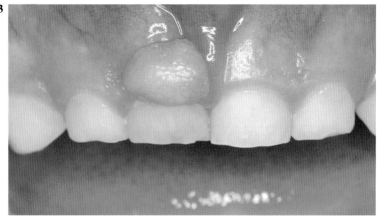

3 (a) What is the lesion above the maxillary primary central incisor?
(b) How did it arise?

4 (a) What abnormality is apparent?
(b) How may the permanent dentition be affected?

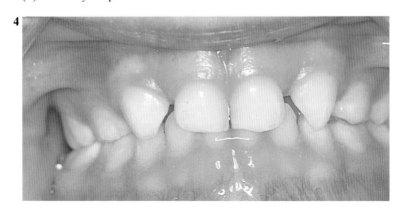

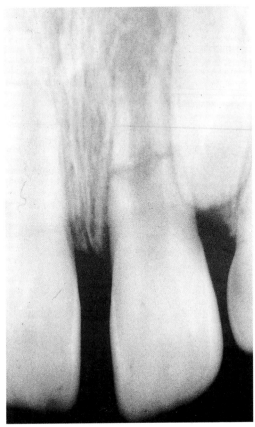

5 (a) What abnormality is shown?
(b) How could it be treated?

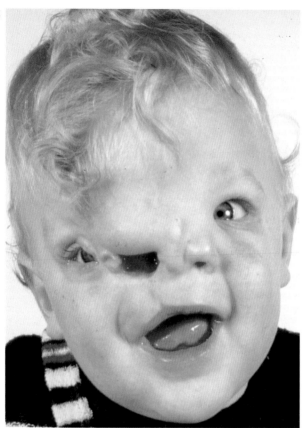

6 What abnormalities affect the face of this baby?

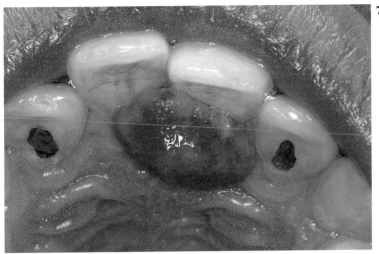

7 This lesion appeared over the preceding four weeks.
(a) What is the diagnosis?
(b) What treatment is required?
(c) How could recurrence be prevented?

8 (a) What are the two abnormalities present?
(b) What is the cause?

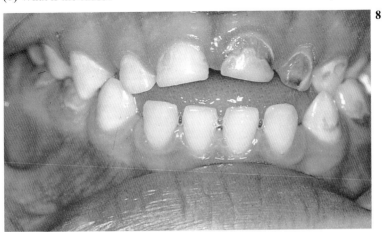

9

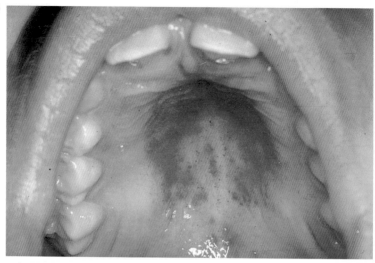

9 (a) What are the palatal lesions in this 11-year-old child?
(b) Of which condition is the appearance suggestive?
(c) How might the diagnosis be confirmed?

10 (a) What has produced the defects on the maxillary central incisors?
(b) At what age did the problem occur?

10

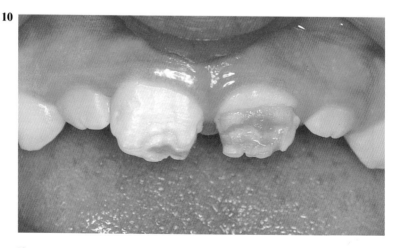

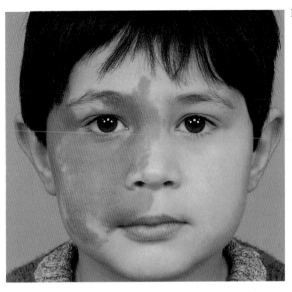

11 (a) What is the diagnosis?
(b) What type of lesion is shown?
(c) What is the significance of the condition to dental treatment?

12 How could the severe discoloration of the two maxillary incisors be treated?

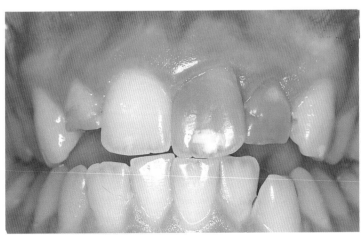

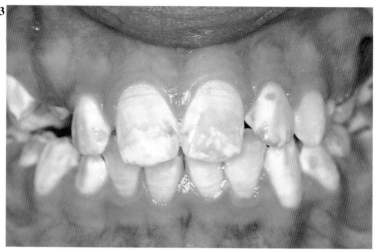

13 (a) What is the diagnosis?
(b) How and where were the defects probably produced?
(c) What treatment is necessary?

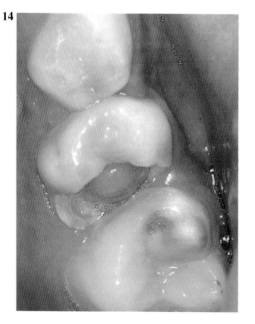

14 (a) What abnormalities are shown?
(b) What treatment is necessary?

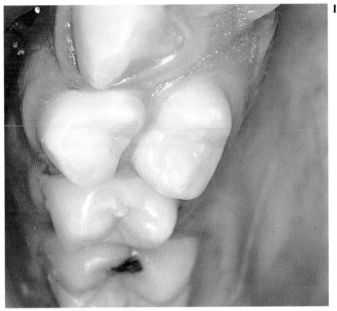

15 (a) Which type of supernumerary tooth is shown?
(b) Where else do these occur?

16 (a) What term is used to describe this skull deformity?
(b) To what group of conditions does it belong?
(c) What is the principal cause of the appearance?

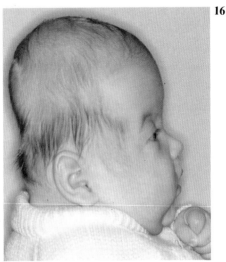

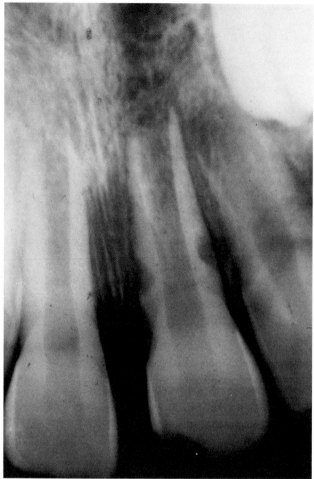

17 (a) What abnormalities are associated with the maxillary left central incisor?
(b) What treatment is indicated?

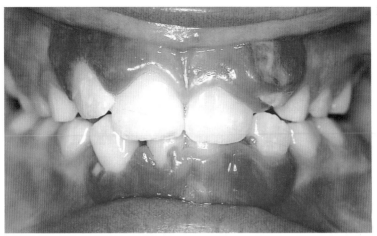

18 This 7-year-old boy has severe periodontal inflammation, particularly around the newly erupted permanent incisors.
(a) What is the differential diagnosis?
(b) How could a diagnosis be confirmed?

19 (a) What abnormality is shown?
(b) How is it transmitted?

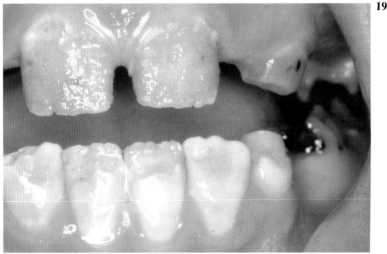

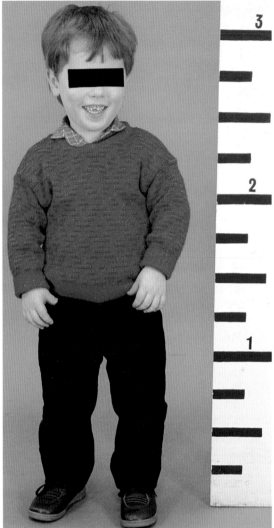

20 (a) What condition affects this 5-year-old, who is small for his age?
(b) What are the typical facial and dental features?
(c) What will be the effect upon his general growth?

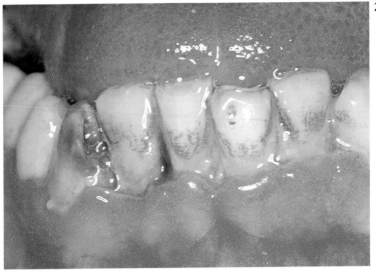

21 (a) What is this periodontal condition?
(b) What factors predispose?
(c) What treatment should be carried out?

22 (a) What is the abnormality?
(b) What complications may arise?
(c) What treatment is indicated?

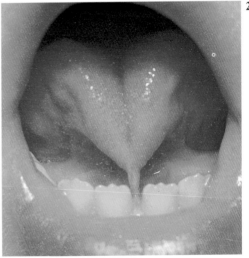

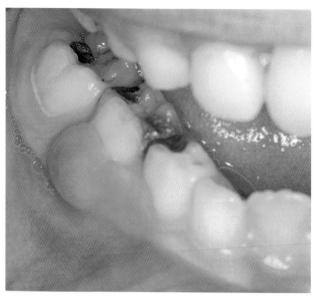

23 (a) What is the cause of this swelling?
(b) How may it be treated?

24 The arm of a 3-year-old girl, reported by her mother to have fallen and damaged her mouth.
(a) What is the lesion?
(b) How should the situation be managed?

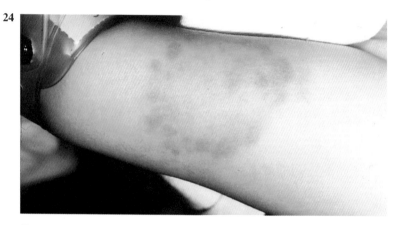

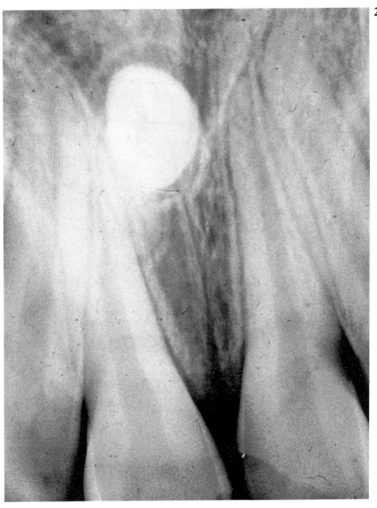

25 (a) What treatment is required for the supernumerary tooth?
(b) What are possible sequelae?

26

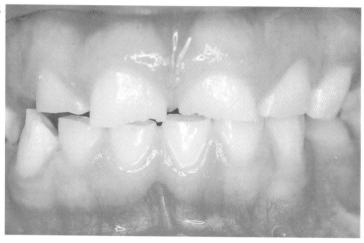

26 (a) What has affected the teeth of this 14-year-old boy?
(b) What are possible causes?
(c) What treatment is required?

27 (a) What name is given to the type of pulp chamber morphology shown particularly well in the maxillary second premolar?
(b) In what condition is it a feature?

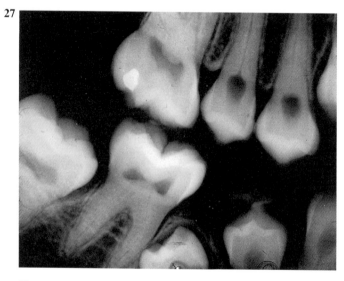

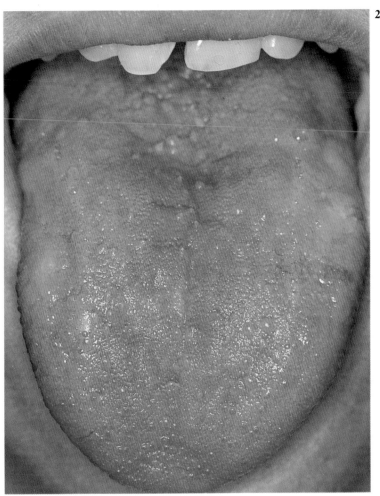

28 A 12-year-old girl has a sore tongue.
(a) What abnormalities are apparent?
(b) What are the possible underlying causes?
(c) Which investigations would assist diagnosis?

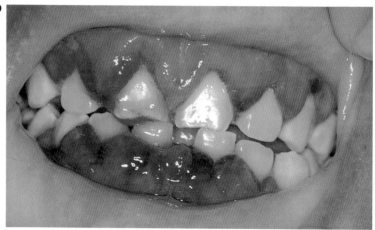

29 This 13-year-old child has severe toothache and swollen, bleeding gums.
(a) What is the possible cause of the gingival condition?
(b) How could the diagnosis be confirmed?
(c) What are the implications for dental treatment?

30 A mother was concerned about the mouth of her three-month-old baby.
(a) What is the condition?
(b) How does it occur?
(c) What treatment is required?

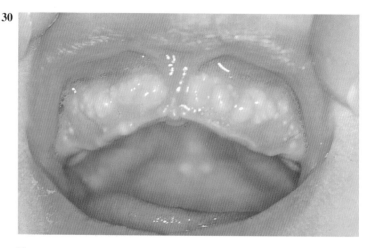

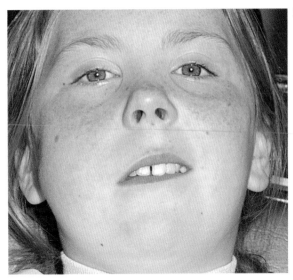

31 The swelling arose within minutes of the infiltration of local anaesthetic solution for restoration of the maxillary right first permanent molar.
(a) What has caused the swelling?
(b) Give three principles of management.

32 (a) What malformation is present on the maxillary right central incisor?
(b) What complications have arisen?
(c) How might these have been prevented?

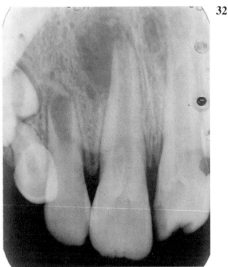

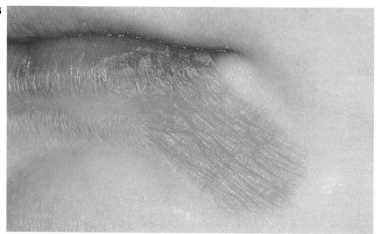

33 This lesion developed two days after pulp therapy to a non-vital primary molar.
(a) What is the lesion?
(b) What should the child's parent be told?
(c) What further action is necessary?

34 (a) What abnormality is shown in this 2-day-old baby?
(b) What treatment is required?
(c) What are possible sequelae?

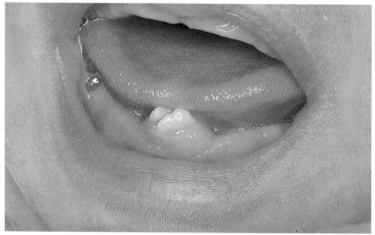

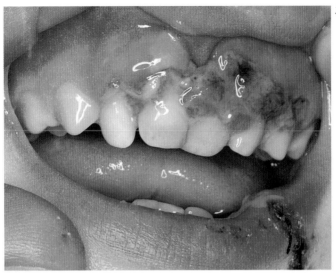

35 This child received trauma some days previously; several teeth are mobile and there is sloughing of associated mucosa. There has been delay in seeking advice. How should the problem be managed?

36 (a) What is this lesion?
(b) What are the characteristic histological features?
(c) What is the treatment and prognosis?

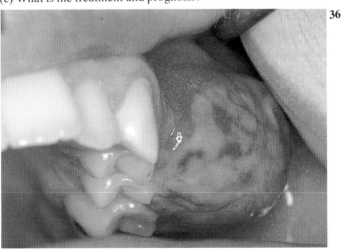

37

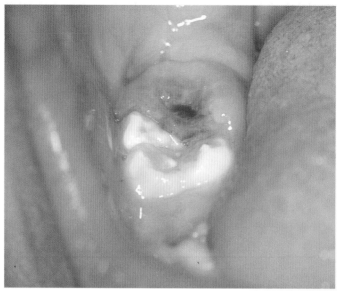

38

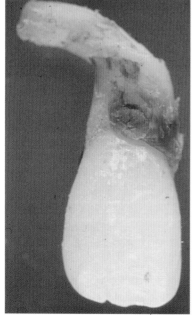

37 (a) What two abnormalities are shown by this 6-year-old child?
(b) How does each arise?
(c) What are the principles of treatment?

38 (a) What is this deformation?
(b) How was it produced?
(c) How old was the child when the defect arose?

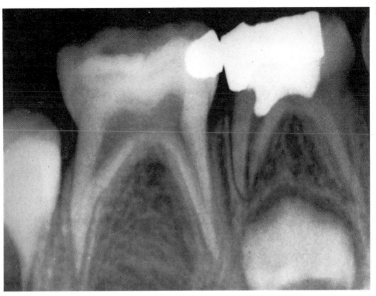

39 (a) What noteworthy features are shown by this radiograph?
(b) How old is the child?
(c) What further investigations are needed?

40 (a) Why have the maxillary permanent central incisors not erupted?
(b) How could the diagnosis be confirmed?
(c) What treatment is needed?

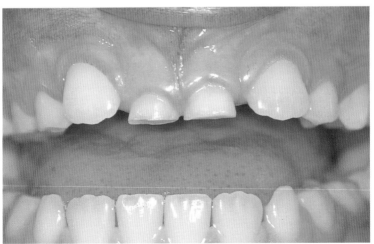

41

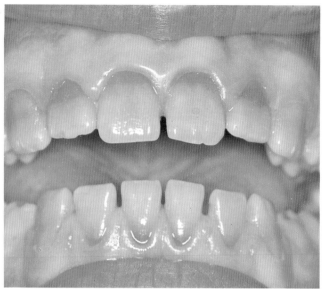

41 (a) What caused the discoloration of these teeth?
(b) What factors determine the nature and extent of the discoloration?
(c) What treatments are available?

42 (a) Why was this radiograph obtained?
(b) What abnormalities are shown?
(c) What treatment is needed?

42

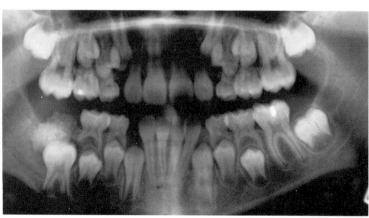

28

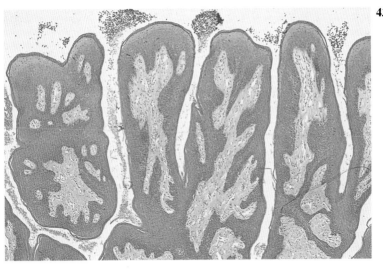

43 (a) What histological features are present on this section from a gingival biopsy?
(b) What is the diagnosis?

44 (a) What abnormality is shown?
(b) What treatment is necessary?

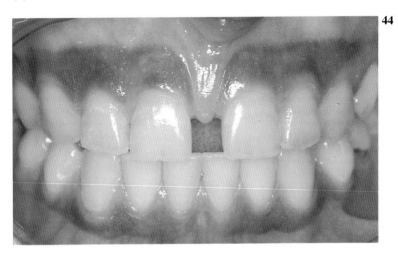

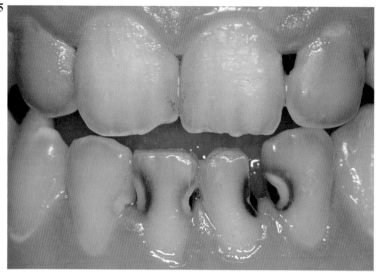

45 (a) Why does this 13-year-old boy have rampant caries?
(b) How may salivary composition affect the distribution of cavities?

46 (a) What is this lesion?
(b) What complications may occur?
(c) What treatment may aid healing?

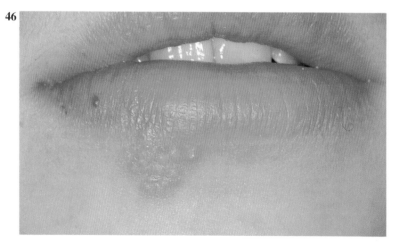

47 (a) What two names are used to describe this malformation?
(b) What treatment is needed?

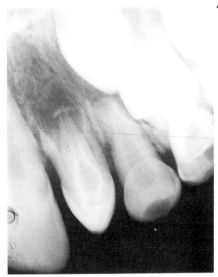

48 (a) What is the lesion on the alveolus?
(b) How could the diagnosis be confirmed?

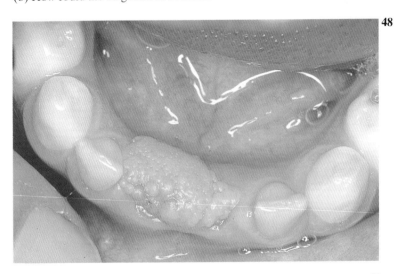

49

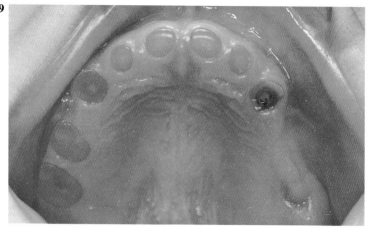

49 This five-year-old girl has gross attrition of the primary teeth.
(a) What is the condition?
(b) How does it arise?

50 (a) What abnormalities are present in this infant's mouth?
(b) What are the principles of treatment?

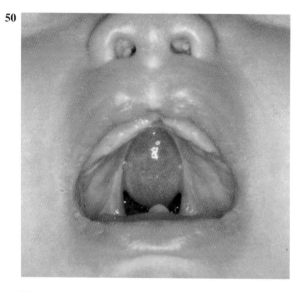

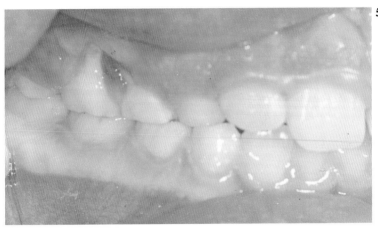

51 (a) What has produced this periodontal appearance?
(b) What is the condition called?
(c) What treatment is required?

52 (a) What abnormality is present on the maxillary left central and lateral incisors?
(b) How does it arise?
(c) What name is given to the nodules on the mandibular incisors?

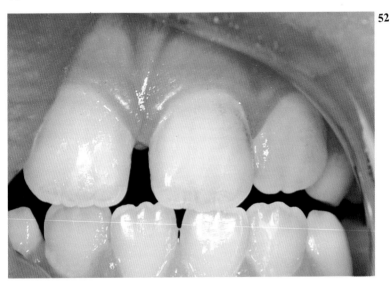

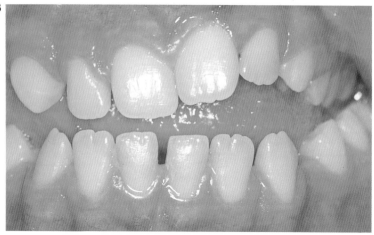

53 (a) What occlusal abnormality is shown?
(b) What is the aetiology?

54 This ground section of dental enamel, seen in polarized light, contains an early carious lesion.
(a) What are the four zones in the lesion?
(b) What does each represent?

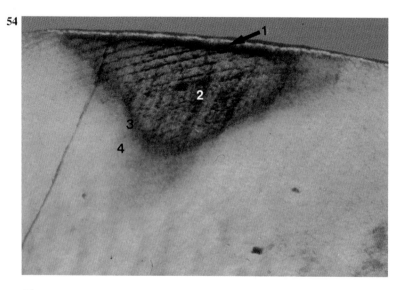

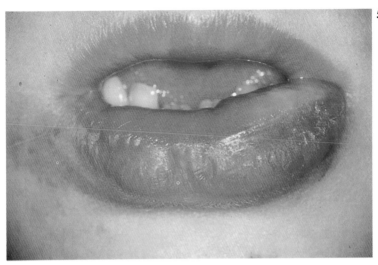

55 This child had a filling placed in the mandibular left quadrant 15 minutes ago.
(a) What has happened?
(b) What treatment is needed?
(c) What other action is required?

56 This 3-year-old received a blow two hours previously which displaced the maxillary primary central incisors palatally.
(a) What treatment is necessary?
(b) What are possible sequelae?

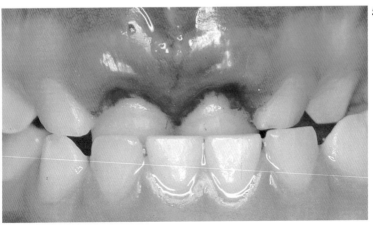

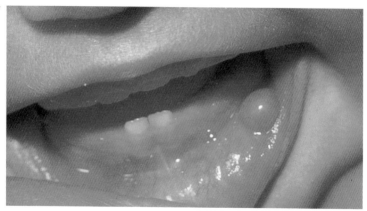

57 (a) What is the lesion on the lower lip?
(b) How did it arise?
(c) What is the treatment?

58 The mother of this 8-year-old child was concerned about the irregularity of the newly erupted teeth.
(a) Which technique will enable treatment to begin immediately?
(b) What is the normal sequence?
(c) What factors must be satisfied before beginning this treatment?

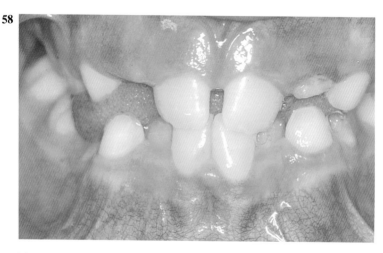

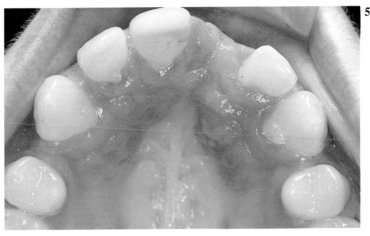

59 A 13-year-old boy is receiving orthodontic treatment.
(a) What has caused this appearance on the palate?
(b) What treatment is necessary?

60 (a) What abnormality is present in this newborn baby?
(b) What are the immediate problems?
(c) How may they be managed?

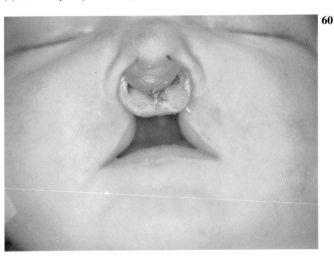

61

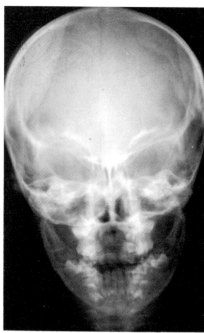

61 (a) What abnormality is shown?
(b) What treatment is required?

62 (a) What abnormality is shown?
(b) How did it arise?
(c) What is the likely consequence to the permanent dentition?

62

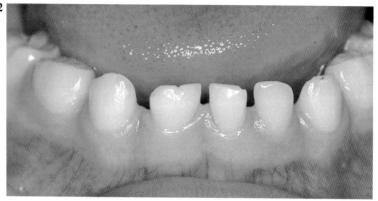

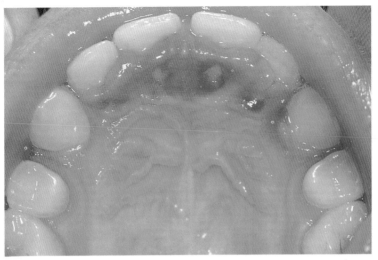

63 (a) What has produced this appearance?
(b) How can the condition be resolved?

64 (a) What is this condition?
(b) What defect enables the achievement of this pose?
(c) What are the characteristic facial features?
(d) What are the associated dental defects?

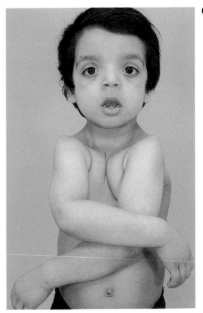

65

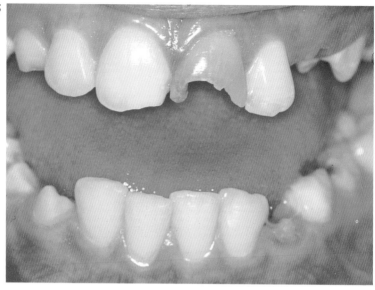

65 This tooth has been on open drainage for several months.
(a) What problems may have arisen?
(b) What initial treatment is needed to save the tooth?
(c) How may the crown be restored in both short and long term?

66

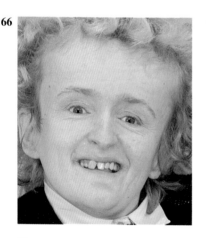

66 (a) What is this condition?
(b) With what other developmental defect is it associated?

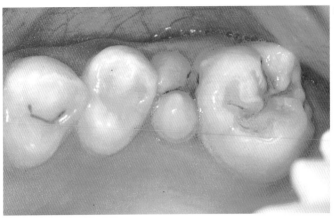

67 (a) Suggest two reasons for this unusual appearance.
(b) What further investigations are required?
(c) What factor would determine possible treatment?

68 (a) What dental abnormalities are shown in this 13-year-old girl?
(b) What are the principles of treatment?
(c) What systemic condition may be associated?

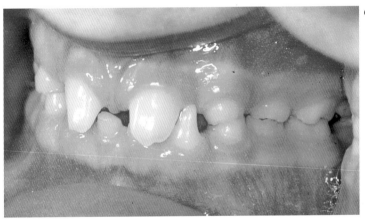

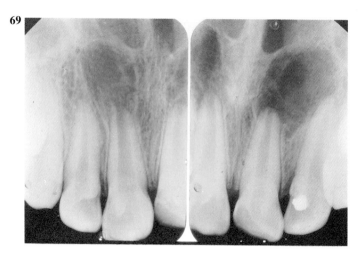

69 This 12-year-old boy damaged his central incisors 3 years ago.
(a) What defects are visible on the radiographs?
(b) How should the teeth be treated?

70 (a) What is the cause of this discoloration?
(b) How did the problem arise?
(c) What treatment is required?

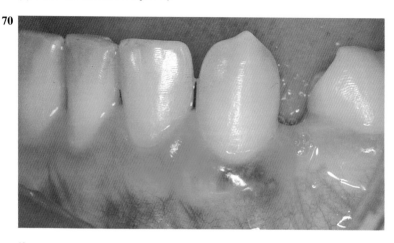

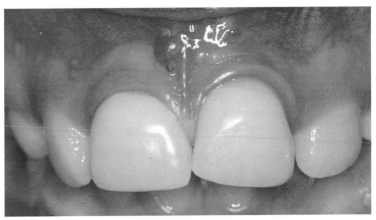

71 An 8-year-old child was fitted with acrylic jacket crowns following the fracture of the maxillary central incisors into enamel and dentine.
(a) What complications have arisen?
(b) What treatment is now indicated?

72 (a) What histological features are shown?
(b) What is the diagnosis?

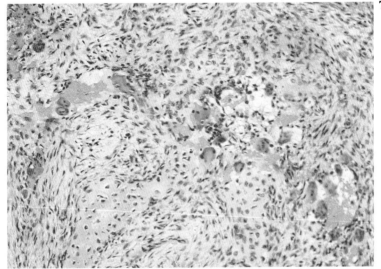

73 (a) What has caused the facial swelling and raised temperature in this 3-year-old girl?
(b) What is a useful intraoral diagnostic sign?

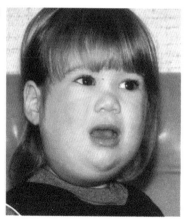

74 (a) What has happened to the second primary molar?
(b) What mechanism is responsible?
(c) What treatment is required?

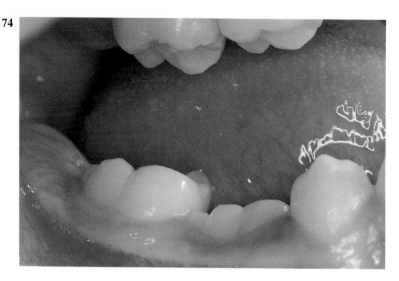

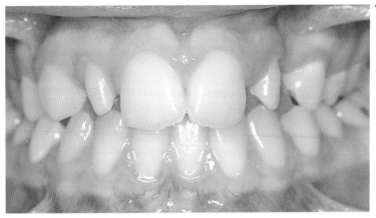

75 What dental anomalies are shown?

76 This 12-year-old boy has a very sore mouth, aggravated by normal toothbrushing. There are bullous skin lesions. Suggest differential diagnoses.

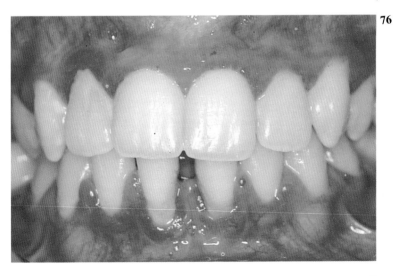

77

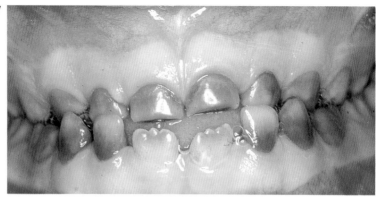

77 (a) What is this condition?
(b) What metabolic defect is responsible?

78 This rash appeared within minutes of a local anaesthetic infiltration. The patient did not feel ill and there was no swelling.
(a) What mechanism produced the rash and what does the appearance represent?
(b) What investigations are needed?

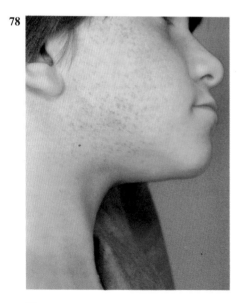

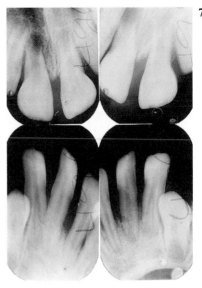

79 The recently erupted incisors of a 7-year-old boy are very mobile. The primary teeth were lost prematurely. Suggest differential diagnoses (nine possible).

80 (a) What condition is shown?
(b) What is the cause?

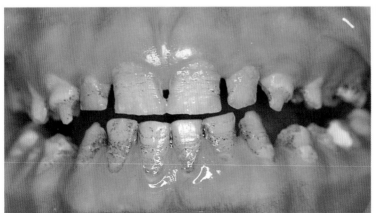

81

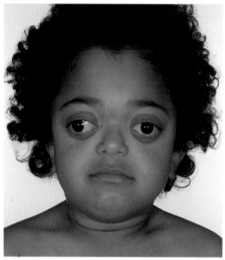

81 (a) What condition is this?
(b) Which features of the condition are visible?
(c) What dental features are commonly associated?

82 (a) What abnormalities are present in this mentally handicapped teenager?
(b) What treatment is necessary?
(c) How could recurrence be minimised?

82

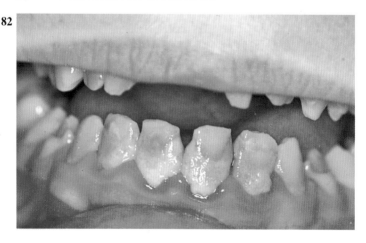

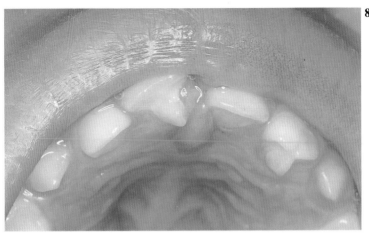

83 (a) What is this unusual tooth morphology?
(b) What problems may it cause?
(c) What treatment is necessary?

84 (a) What is this appliance?
(b) What is the strongest indication for its use?

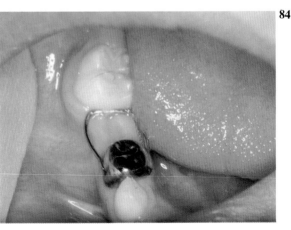

85

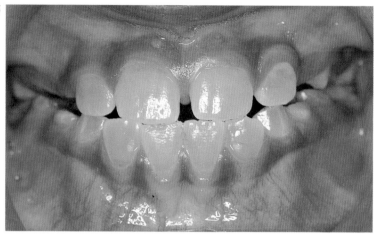

85 (a) What are the two names for this condition?
(b) What problems are likely?

86

86 (a) What defects are shown in this congenital condition?
(b) To what group does the condition belong?
(c) What is the specific defect in this child?

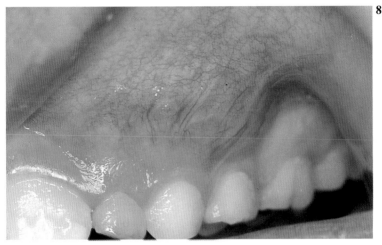

87, 88 (a) What is this condition?
(b) What complications may arise?
(c) What treatment is necessary?

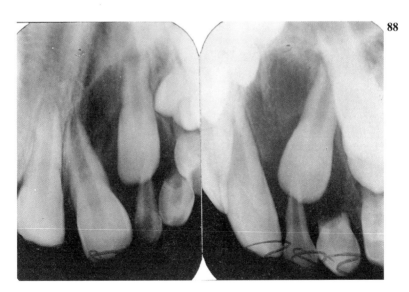

89

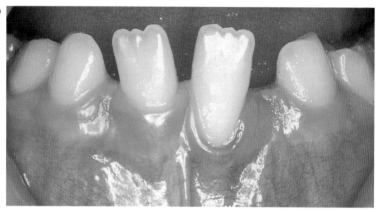

89 (a) What condition is associated with the mandibular left central incisor?
(b) How did it arise?
(c) What treatment is necessary?

90 (a) What is the most likely diagnosis?
(b) Which tests would confirm this?
(c) What is the treatment?

90

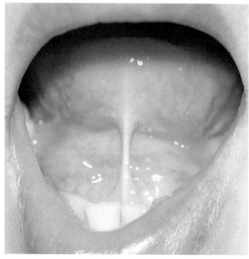

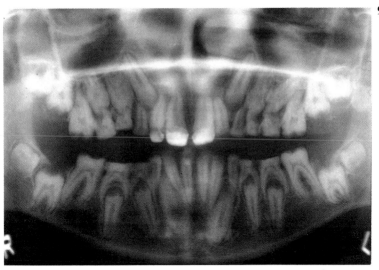

91 (a) What abnormalities are apparent on the panoral radiograph of this 15-year-old boy?
(b) What factors may be responsible?

92 This 3-year-old girl was asked to show her teeth.
(a) What is wrong?
(b) Suggest a differential diagnosis.

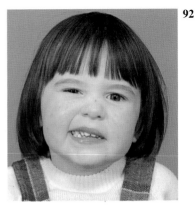

93 (a) What condition has caused this discoloration?
(b) What treatment is necessary?

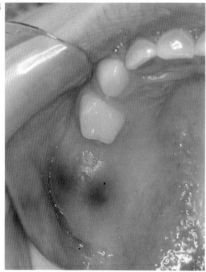

94 (a) What abnormalities are visible in this 9-year-old child?
(b) What factors may have contributed to the problem?
(c) What treatment is necessary?

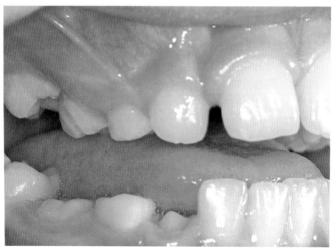

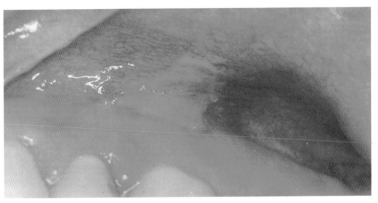

95 This mucosal lesion was present following conservative work in the area.
(a) What is the diagnosis?
(b) How can recurrence be avoided?

96 (a) What is adjacent to the lingual fraenum?
(b) What symptoms may arise?
(c) What treatment is indicated?
(d) What further tests should be made?

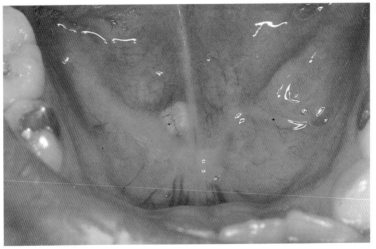

97

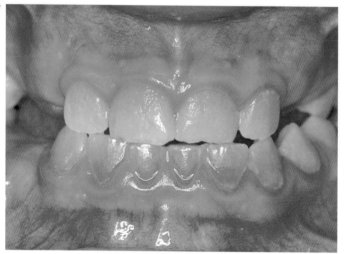

97 (a) Suggest two possible causes for this dental appearance.
(b) What features of the history and examination would help to establish the diagnosis?
(c) Which special test would confirm it?

98 This seven-year-old girl and her sister both had swollen, red, ulcerated gums.
(a) What is the diagnosis?
(b) How is the condition transmitted?
(c) What treatment is needed?

98

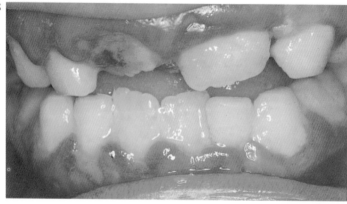

99 (a) What abnormalities are shown?
(b) What is the condition?
(c) How is it transmitted?

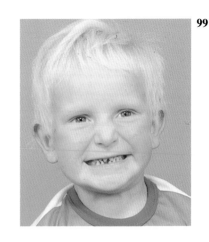

100 (a) What name is given to the malformation of the second premolar?
(b) What is the cause?

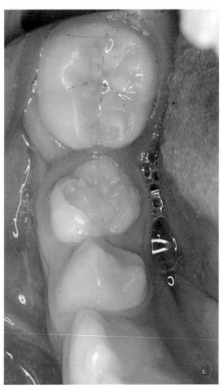

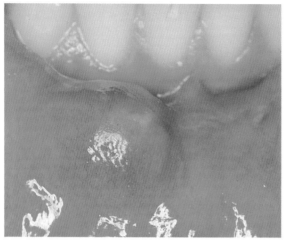

101 (a) What has caused the swelling?
(b) What is the lesion?
(c) Where may this type of lesion occur?

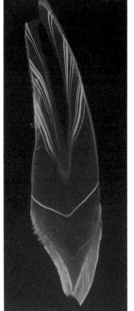

102 (a) What has produced the fluorescent
bands in this tooth section?
(b) What is the mechanism?
(c) What is the clinical effect?

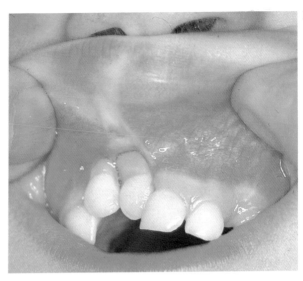

103 (a) What has produced the periodontal destruction in this three-year-old child?
(b) What are the dental effects of the condition?
(c) What are the histological findings?

104 (a) What is this syndrome?
(b) Which of the main features are visible?
(c) What is a possible anaesthetic hazard in this condition?

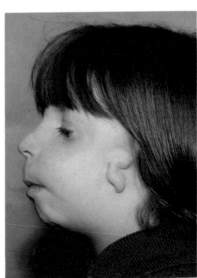

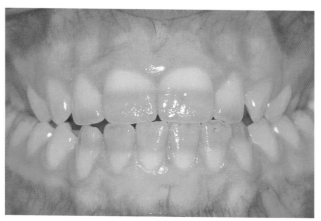

105 This child received prolonged tetracycline therapy.
(a) What effect has this produced?
(b) What systemic condition used to be treated by prolonged tetracycline therapy?

106 (a) Which type of supernumerary tooth is this?
(b) What other supernumerary elements occur in the premaxilla?

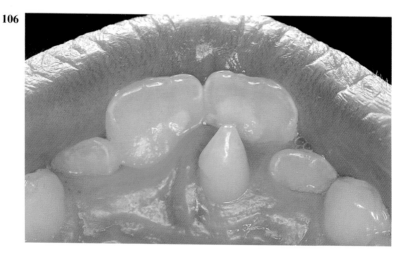

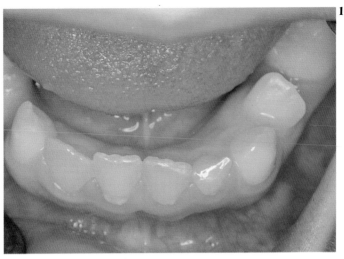

107 (a) What unusual feature is shown?
(b) How did it arise?

108 (a) What has produced this appearance?
(b) How might the condition be resolved?

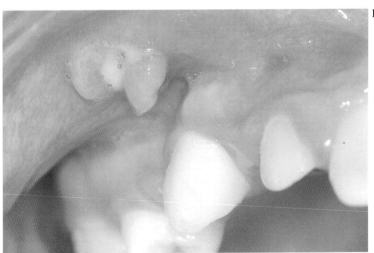

109 This girl has just fallen from her bicycle.
(a) What local treatment do her injuries require?
(b) What systemic treatment is indicated?

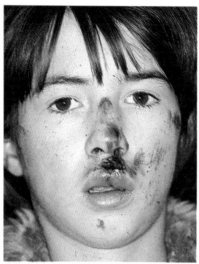

110 (a) What is the lesion in the sulcus?
(b) What further investigations are indicated?
(c) With what systemic conditions might the ulcer be associated?

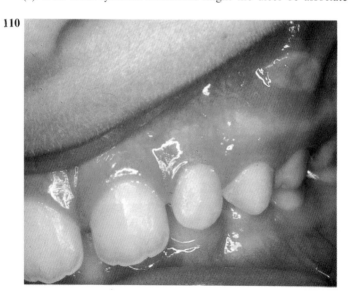

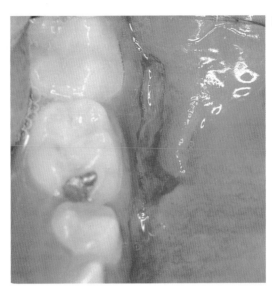

111,112 The cheeks and swollen lips of a 10-year-old boy who suffers recurrent oral ulcers associated with hyperplastic ridges.
(a) What is the condition?
(b) What test confirms the diagnosis?
(c) How is the condition treated?

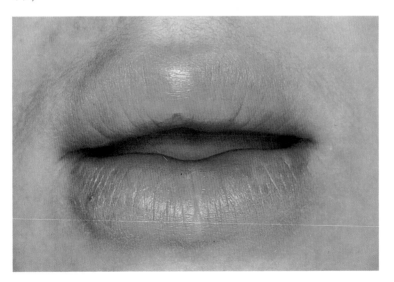

113

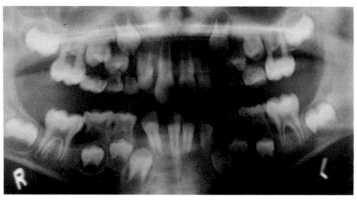

113 (a) What abnormalities are shown on the panoral radiograph of this seven-year-old child?
(b) What further investigations would aid diagnosis?
(c) What condition is suggested?

114 (a) What has produced this enamel hypoplasia?
(b) What name is given to the condition?
(c) What are the typical features?

114

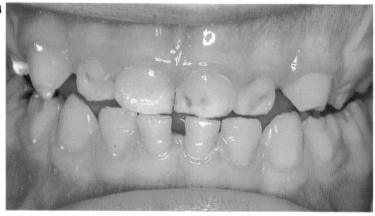

115 This six-year-old girl has no history of trauma.
(a) What is the condition?
(b) What are the characteristic features?
(c) What is the aetiological mechanism?

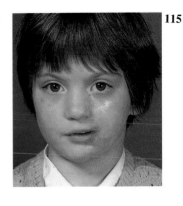

115

116 (a) What morphological and histological malformations are present on this maxillary primary incisor?
(b) What condition is represented?

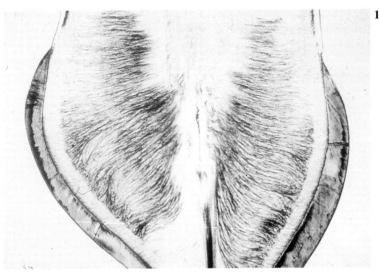

116

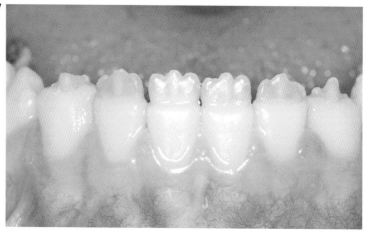

117 This girl thrived as a baby until she was introduced to solid food.
(a) At what age was she weaned?
(b) What systemic condition was then manifested?
(c) What other teeth are likely to be affected?

118 (a) What problems are present in this 3-year-old child?
(b) What treatment is needed?
(c) What advice should be given to the parent?

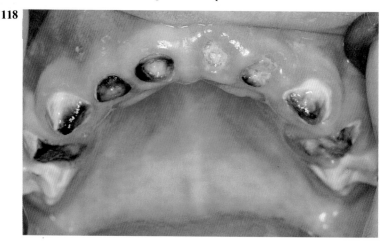

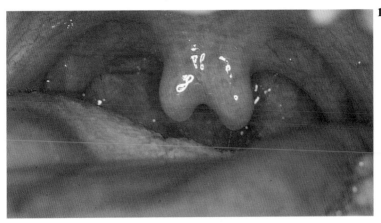

119 What abnormalities may be associated with this bifid uvula?

120 (a) How old is this child?
(b) Suggest 5 causes for the median diastema.

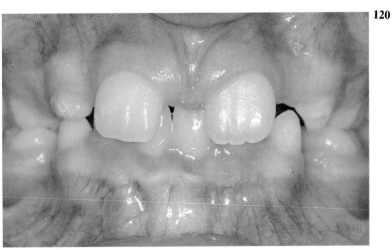

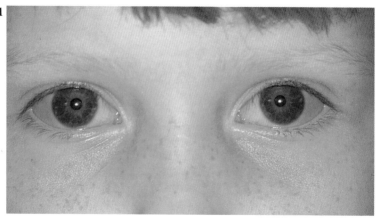

121 (a) Which condition has this ocular appearance as a diagnostic feature?
(b) How is this appearance produced?
(c) What dental condition may be associated?

122 (a) What has produced discoloration of the tongue and teeth in this mentally retarded teenage girl?
(b) How may staining be avoided?

122

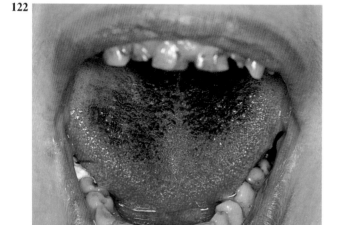

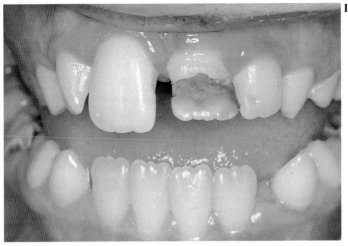

123 The tip of the left central incisor is labially inclined.
(a) How was the defect produced?
(b) At what age did the damage occur?
(c) What is the treatment?

124 The maxillary right central incisor was traumatized 2 years ago.
(a) What sequence of events has produced this appearance?
(b) What are the treatment possibilities?

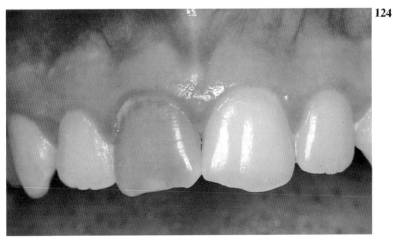

125

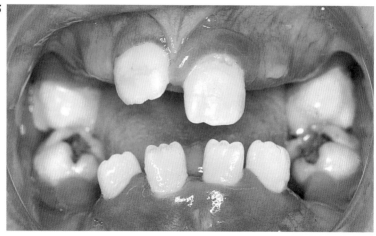

125 This 7-year-old Asian boy has palmar skin that is thickened and fissured. Several primary teeth exfoliated prematurely before the rest were extracted. All permanent teeth are now mobile.
(a) What is the condition?
(b) How is it managed?

126

126 (a) What is this condition?
(b) What are the typical facial features?
(c) How is it transmitted?

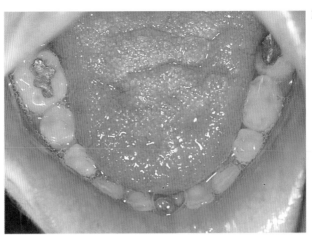

127 (a) What abnormalities are present on this tongue?
(b) What condition is suggested?
(c) What problems may arise?
(d) How may they be avoided?

128 (a) What abnormality is present?
(b) How does it arise?
(c) What treatment is advisable?

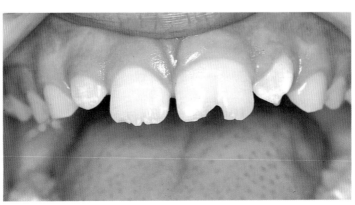

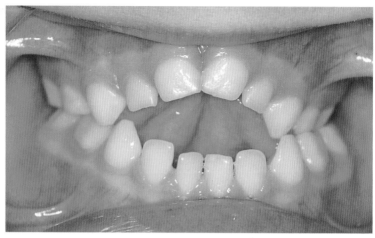

129 (a) What abnormalities are shown?
(b) How did they arise?
(c) Are the defects likely to persist?

130 This patient has Hodgkin's disease.
(a) What is the lesion in this condition?
(b) What is the characteristic histological finding?
(c) What has happened to the teeth?

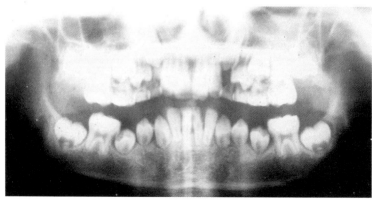

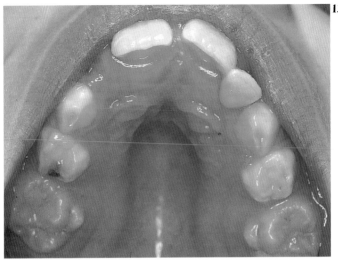

131 Extraction of the maxillary second primary molars has produced marked space loss.
(a) What 3 factors will have influenced the rate and extent of loss?
(b) Which have greater mesio-distal dimensions: the primary canine and two primary molars or the permanent canine and two premolars?
(c) What is the difference called?

132 A fluoride-containing varnish is being applied.
(a) What is the usual concentration of fluoride salt in a varnish?
(b) What level of fluoride ion does this represent?

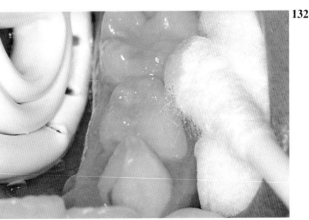

132

133

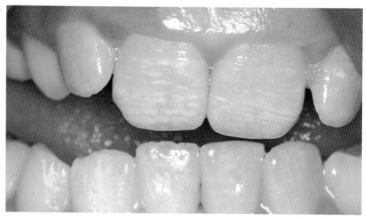

133 (a) What has produced this dental appearance?
(b) What features support the diagnosis?

134 These natal teeth are very firm.
(a) What problem may they cause?
(b) What is the treatment?

134

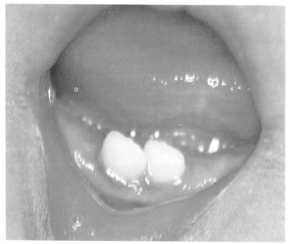

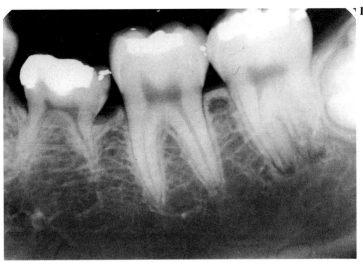

135 (a) What dental abnormalities are shown?
(b) What treatment is indicated?
(c) What factors support this plan?

136 (a) What has caused the tooth discoloration?
(b) At what stage was the agent active?
(c) How could the diagnosis be confirmed?

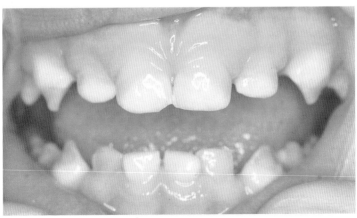

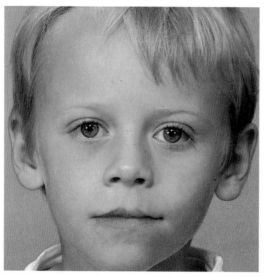

137 The face of this 8-year-old boy developed normally until 5 years of age.
(a) What abnormalities are now apparent?
(b) What further investigations are needed?
(c) What is the probable diagnosis?

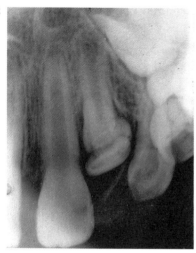

138 There is a history of trauma to the maxillary primary lateral incisor.
(a) What abnormality is present?
(b) When did the accident occur?
(c) What mechanism produces this type of damage?

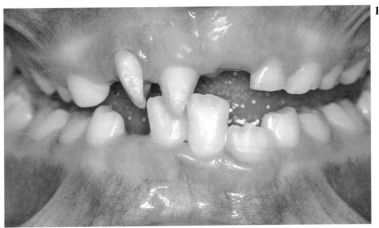

139 (a) What abnormality is shown?
(b) What are the typical morphological features?
(c) What is the most common site for supernumerary teeth?

140 This child fell 2 hours ago and intruded 3 incisors.
(a) What treatment is required for the 3 recently intruded teeth?
(b) How would the problem be managed in the intermediate term?

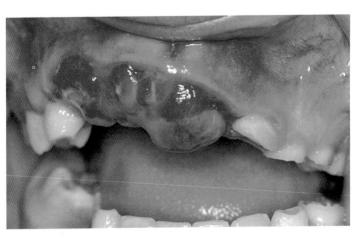

141

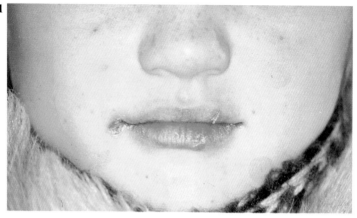

141 A child has recurrent facial lesions of this type.
(a) What is the condition?
(b) What is the cause?
(c) How is the condition transmitted?

142 This tooth was fractured into dentine two weeks previously.
(a) What investigations are required?
(b) What is the immediate treatment?

142

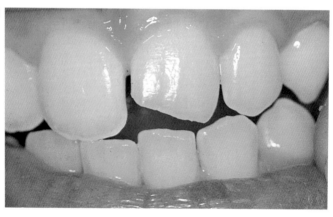

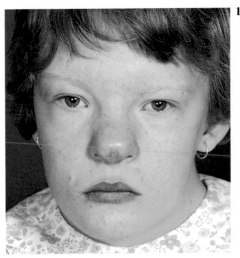

143 This 14-year-old girl is distressed by light exercise.
(a) What is unusual about her appearance?
(b) Suggest the underlying cause.
(c) How does this affect dental treatment?

144 A 12-year-old child was receiving orthodontic treatment to approximate the maxillary central incisors.
(a) What abnormality is shown?
(b) What is the cause?

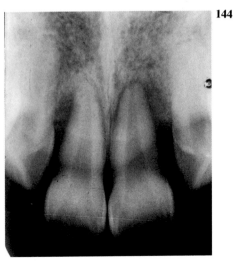

145

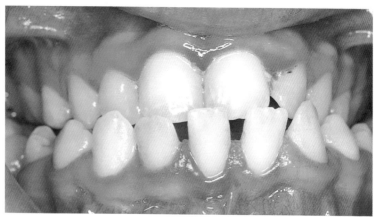

145 What dental features, typical of Down's syndrome, are illustrated?

146 (a) What facial abnormalities are apparent in this 15-year-old girl?
(b) What syndrome is this?
(c) What are the associated dental problems?

146

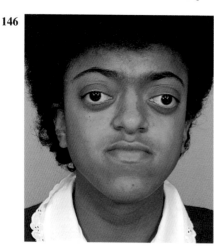

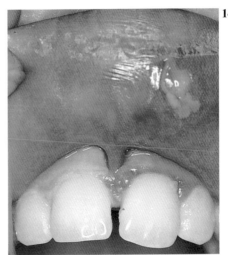

147 The maxillary left central incisor was hit by an airgun pellet the previous day and is very mobile.
(a) What investigations are required?
(b) What dental treatment is needed?

148 (a) What is this skin condition?
(b) What is the dental implication?
(c) What is the underlying defect?

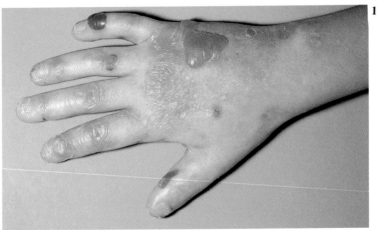

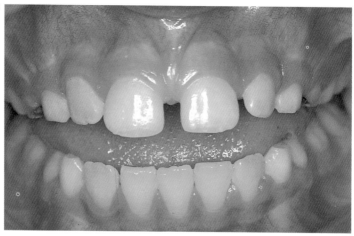

149 (a) What features are shown?
(b) What treatment is needed?

150 (a) What dental abnormality is apparent in this girl?
(b) What hypothesis describes the production of this particular form?
(c) What are the likely complaints of the patient?

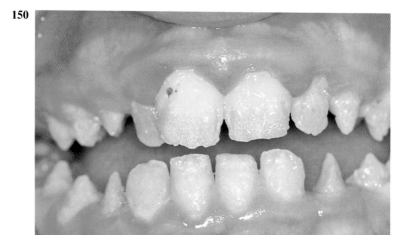

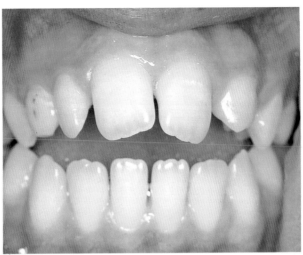

151 (a) What is the most probable cause of this anterior open bite?
(b) What other signs are frequently associated with this condition?

152 (a) What is this periodontal condition?
(b) What treatment is needed?
(c) How may recurrence be prevented?

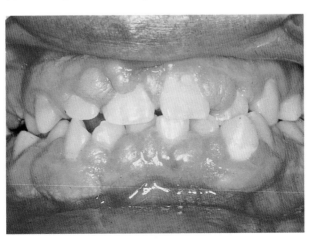

153

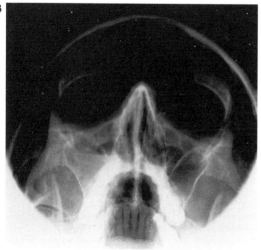

153 A 15-year-old patient complained of pain in the maxillary right molar teeth.
(a) What radiographic view is shown?
(b) What radiographic appearance suggests a diagnosis for the pain?
(c) What treatment is necessary?

154

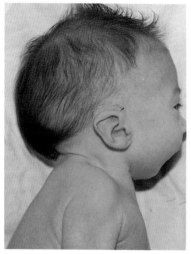

154 (a) What is this condition?
(b) What is the most important feature of early management?
(c) What is the prognosis?

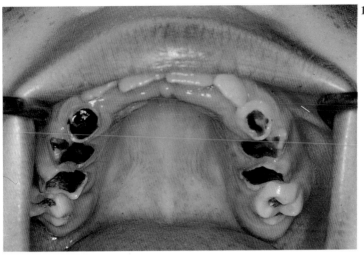

155 (a) What condition is present in the mouth of this 8-year-old child?
(b) What is the cause?
(c) What treatment is indicated?

156 (a) What is the white area on the alveolus?
(b) What is the cause?

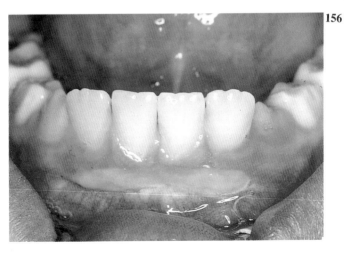

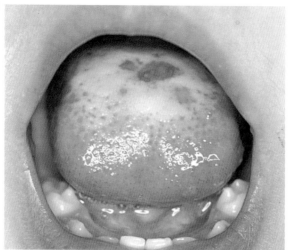

157 This 2-year-old child is unwell and has itchy hands and feet.
(a) What is the cause?
(b) What is the treatment?

158 (a) What is this condition?
(b) How did it arise?

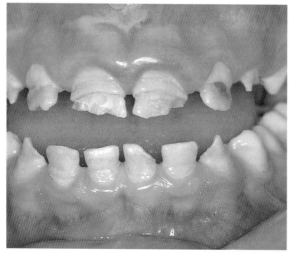

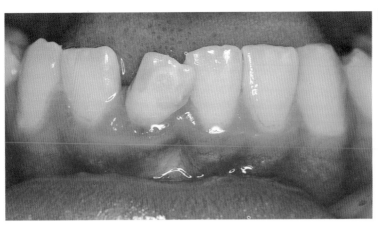

159 (a) What abnormalities are apparent on the mandibular right central incisor?
(b) How were they caused?

160 (a) Suggest two diagnoses.
(b) What treatment is required?
(c) What is the prognosis?

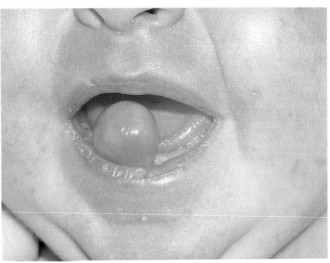

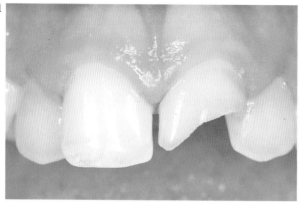

161 An 8-year-old child fractured the maxillary left central incisor two months ago with pulpal involvement. This tooth is non-vital.
(a) What was the correct emergency treatment at the time of injury?
(b) What treatment is now required?
(c) What medicaments are specifically contra-indicated?

162 (a) What dental abnormality is present in this 13-year-old girl?
(b) How did it arise?
(c) What treatment is necessary?

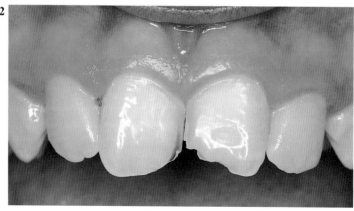

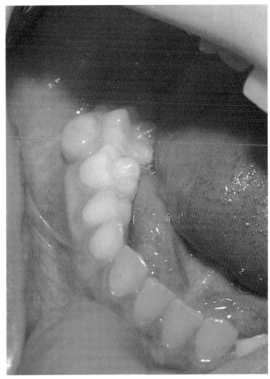

163 This rapidly enlarging swelling was first noticed 3 weeks previously.
(a) What is the most significant associated feature?
(b) What treatment is required?
(c) Suggest differential diagnoses.

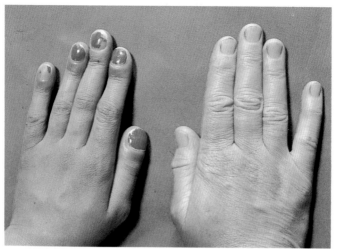

164 The left hand belongs to a girl with Fallot's tetralogy, the right hand is normal.
(a) What physical signs are present on the left hand?
(b) What are the components of Fallot's tetralogy?

165 (a) What is the quadrilateral area in this neonatal skull?
(b) At what age should it close?

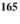

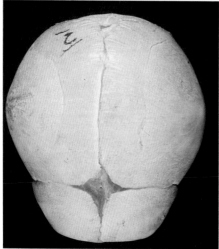

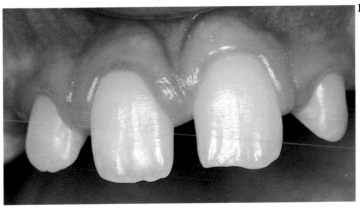

166 (a) What name is given to this stage of occlusal development?
(b) How is the appearance produced?

167 (a) What are shown on this scanning electronmicrograph?
(b) What agent is usually employed to produce this effect?

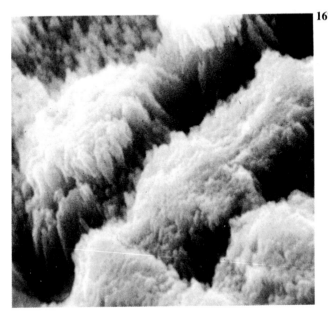

168

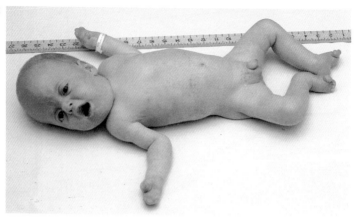

168 (a) What condition is this?
(b) What diagnostic abnormalities are visible?

169 (a) Identify these teeth.
(b) What are likely sequelae in the permanent dentition?

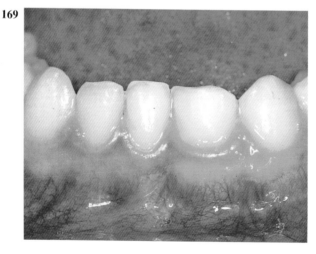

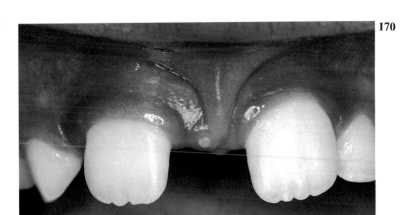

170 (a) What is the cause of this midline diastema?
(b) What treatment is necessary at this stage?

171 (a) What is this intracranial device?
(b) In what condition is it used?
(c) What structures does it connect?

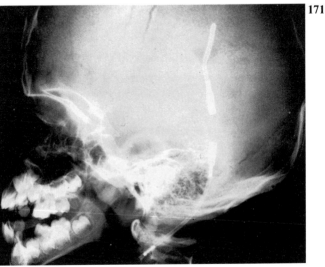

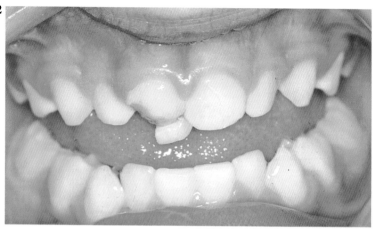

172 This 4-year-old child fractured the maxillary primary central incisor some hours previously. The fracture line extends subgingivally and the pulp is exposed.
(a) What is the treatment?
(b) What are the possible sequelae?

173 (a) What defects affect the lower incisors?
(b) How did they arise?
(c) At what age did this occur?

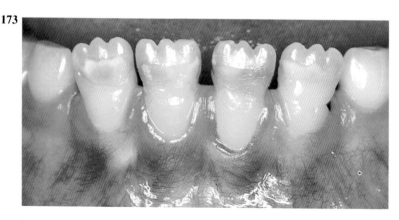

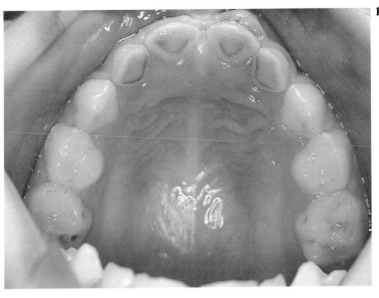

174 (a) What abnormalities are shown?
(b) What is the most likely cause?

175 (a) What has caused the white line on the cheek mucosa?
(b) What action is required?

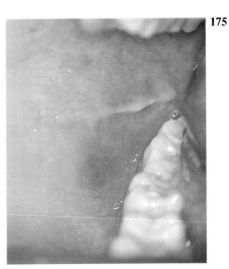

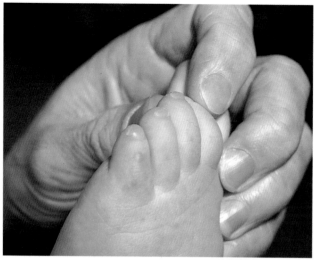

176 (a) What lesions are shown on the foot of this 3-year-old child?
(b) Similar lesions are present in the mouth; what is the condition?
(c) What is the cause?

177 (a) What agent has produced this appearance?
(b) What mechanism is involved?
(c) How may the problem be minimised?

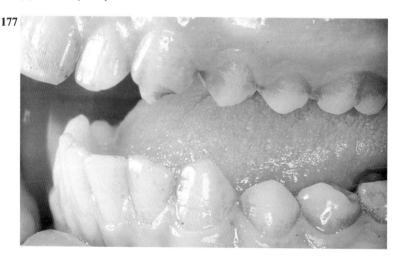

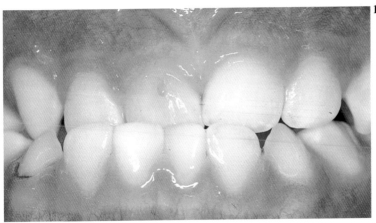

178 (a) What condition affects the maxillary right primary central incisor?
(b) How is it produced?
(c) What treatment is required?

179 A 4-year-old child had a supplemental maxillary primary lateral incisor that was exfoliated.
(a) What physical signs are now present?
(b) What investigations would assist diagnosis?
(c) What is the diagnosis?

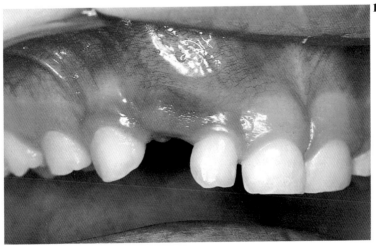

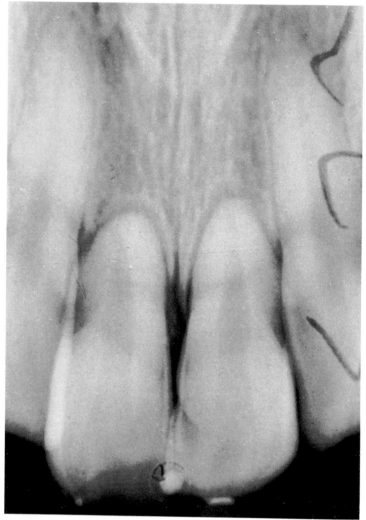

180 This 12-year-old child suffered a blow 2 years ago with resultant tooth mobility.
(a) What has happened?
(b) What is the prognosis?
(c) What treatment is indicated?

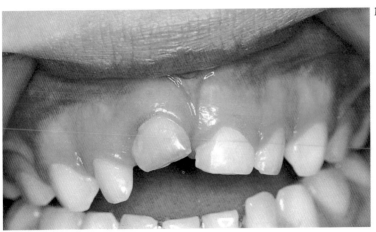

181 The maxillary primary central incisor was intruded by a fall 1 year previously.
(a) What has occurred?
(b) What later sequelae may follow this type of injury?

182 A 9-month-old infant is fretful and has a rash on her left cheek.
(a) What is the significance of the rash?
(b) How may the condition be treated?

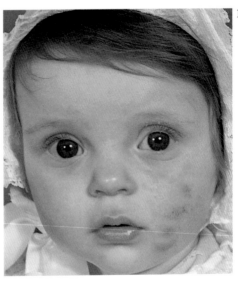

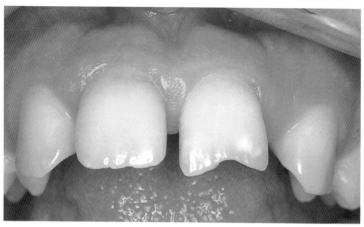

183 (a) What 4 dental abnormalities are shown?
(b) Suggest the cause of each.

184 (a) How old is this child?
(b) What is the diagnosis?
(c) What treatment is required?

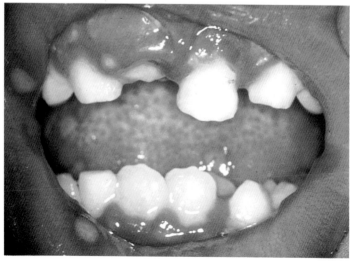

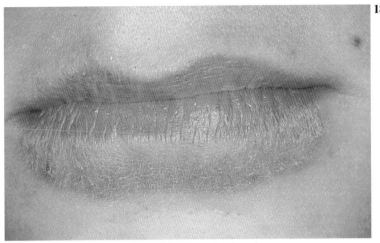

185 (a) What is this appearance called?
(b) How does it arise?
(c) What treatment is required?

186 (a) What is the diagnosis?
(b) What is the prognosis?
(c) What principle governs dental treatment?

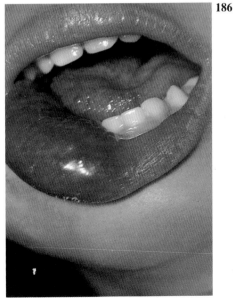

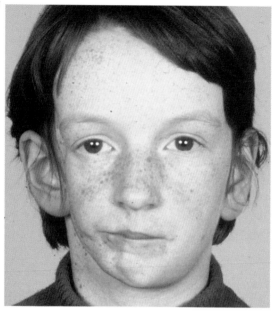

187 This 13-year-old boy developed normally until he was 5 years old.
(a) What condition is now apparent?
(b) What is the characteristic appearance and how is it produced?
(c) What neurological conditions may be associated?

188 (a) What abnormality is this?
(b) What treatment would be helpful?

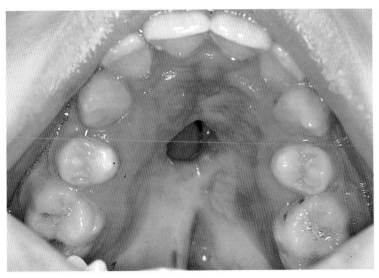

189 (a) What conditions are shown?
(b) What treatment is necessary?

190 This child has very large teeth in the premaxilla and the right lateral incisor is missing.
(a) How did this occur?
(b) What features of the condition will affect management?

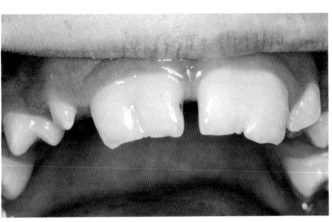

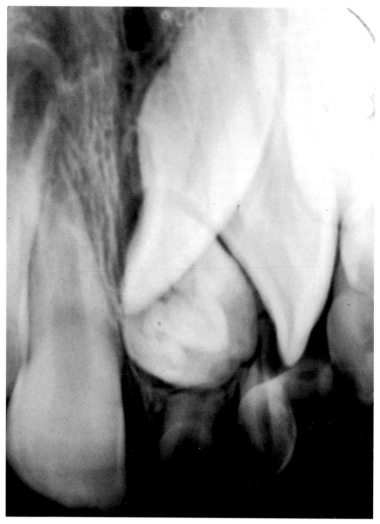

191 What abnormalities are shown?

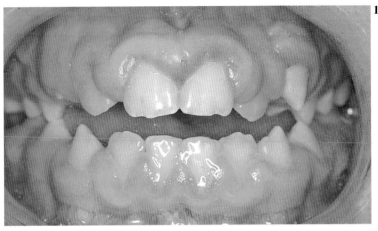

192 (a) What is the cause of the gingival appearance?
(b) By what mechanism is the swelling produced?
(c) What treatment is needed?

193 (a) What is the diagnosis?
(b) How does the lesion arise?
(c) What is the long-term effect?

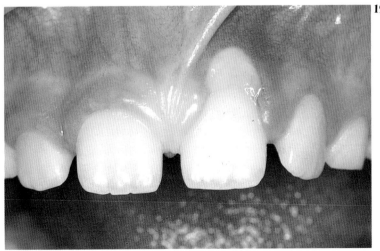

194

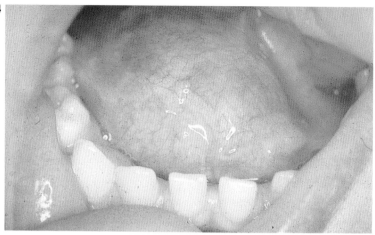

194 A 7-year-old boy has a sublingual swelling which is causing problems with speech and swallowing.
(a) What is the lesion?
(b) What is the differential diagnosis?
(c) How would the diagnosis be confirmed?
(d) Where is the lesion situated?

195 This severely mentally handicapped teenager has spastic cerebral palsy and aggressive self-mutilating behaviour.
(a) What is the condition?
(b) What underlying defect is responsible?
(c) How may further trauma be avoided?

195

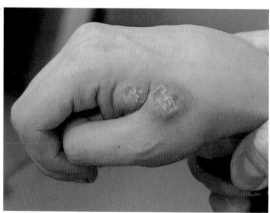

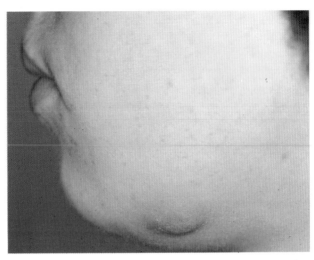

196 The teeth of this 10-year-old child have been neglected. There had been submandibular swelling for 3 weeks.
(a) What is the differential diagnosis?
(b) Outline a programme of management.

197 A panoramic radiograph shows features pathognomic of a dental condition.
(a) What are the abnormalities?
(b) What is the condition?

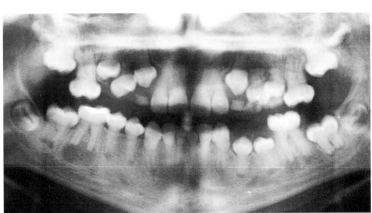

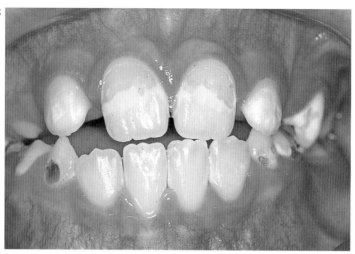

198 (a) What has caused the appearance of the maxillary teeth?
(b) What further investigation is necessary?
(c) What treatment is required?

199 (a) What name is given to this marked type of facial asymmetry?
(b) How does it arise?
(c) What dental problems are associated?

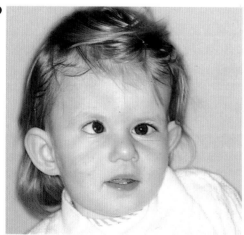

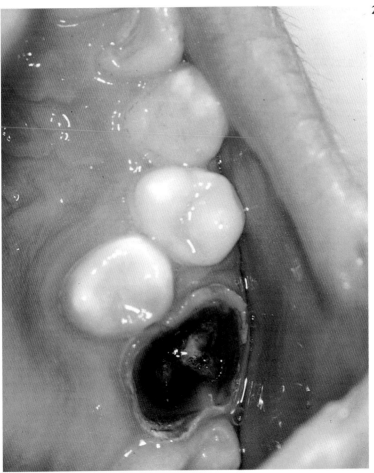

200 (a) What two dental problems are present?
(b) What is the common aetiology?
(c) What treatment is required?

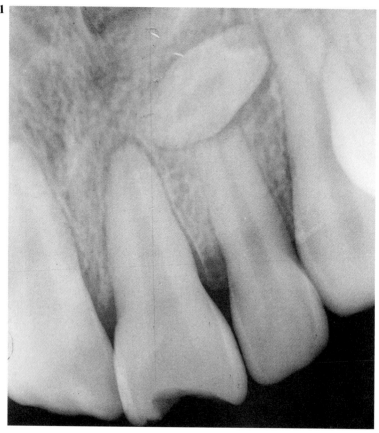

201 (a) What abnormalities are shown?
(b) What treatment is indicated?

ANSWERS

1 (a) Alveolar fracture.
(b) Orthodontic realignment. Manual repositioning is contra-indicated since the teeth are now firm and vital.

2 (a) Lip repair at 3 months, palate repair between 6 months and 1 year.
(b) Hypodontia; hypoplastic teeth; Class III malocclusion with bilateral cross bite.

3 (a) Fibro-epithelial polyp.
(b) Exuberant reaction to chronic infection from a non-vital pulp.

4 (a) Missing maxillary primary lateral incisors.
(b) Missing maxillary lateral incisors; increased incidence of other missing teeth.

5 (a) Root fracture in the middle third.
(b) Cement splint and leave for two months in an attempt to induce repair at the fracture line. Later treatment may include endodontics with the use of full length silver point to splint root fragments.

6 Unilateral facial cleft; encephalocoele; hypertelorism.

7 (a) Exuberant inflammation following repeated trauma to the incisive papilla.
(b) Excision biopsy.
(c) By preventing further trauma to the palate.

8 (a) Anterior open bite; labial caries.
(b) Prolonged use of a comforter bottle or dipped dummy.

9 (a) Petechial haemorrhages.
(b) Infectious mononucleosis (glandular fever).
(c) Other signs include fever and generalised lymphadenopathy. Specific blood tests are definitive e.g. Monospot test.

10 (a) Trauma to primary central incisors with intrusion of the left one.
(b) 6-9 months; the maxillary permanent central incisors commence crown calcification at 3-4 months post-natally.

11 (a) Capillary haemangioma.
(b) Hamartoma (a tumour-like developmental defect).
(c) If the lesion involves bone, extractions may produce uncontrollable haemorrhage.

12 Endodontics; attempt bleaching procedure; composite or porcelain veneers; post crowns.

13 (a) Severe fluorosis.
(b) By drinking well water in the Indian subcontinent.
(c) Composite or porcelain veneers.

14 (a) Pulp polyp maxillary second primary molar; hypoplasia of first permanent molar.
(b) Extract maxillary second primary molar; consider space maintenance; restore first permanent molar.

15 (a) A supplemental tooth.
(b) In the maxillary lateral incisor and third molar regions; more rarely in the mandibular incisor region.

16 (a) Turricephaly (turret skull).
(b) The craniosynostoses.
(c) Premature fusion of skull sutures. In this child the coronal and lambdoid sutures are involved.

17 (a) Crown fracture; arrested root development; external resorption; pulp death.
(b) Endodontic therapy using calcium hydroxide to combat external resorption and induce an apical barrier.

18 (a) Prepubertal periodontitis, alone or associated with a systemic factor; scleroderma; diabetes; hyperparathyroidism; Cushing's disease; Histiocytosis-X; Papillon-Lefèvre syndrome. In this case the diagnosis was Histiocytosis-X.
(b) Biopsy; haematology; immunology.

19 (a) Amelogenesis imperfecta (hypocalcified type).
(b) Autosomal dominance is usual. However, the method of inheritance varies and forms the basis of classification.

20 (a) Achondroplasia.
(b) Large head; frontal bossing; depressed nose; maxillary hypoplasia; class III malocclusion.
(c) Early closure of epiphyses will result in restricted growth of long bones.

21 (a) Acute ulcerative gingivitis.
(b) Poor oral hygiene and calculus; smoking; stress and reduced general resistance.
(c) Oral hygiene; scaling; débridement; prescribe metronidazole.

22 (a) Ankyloglossia.
(b) Impaired oral cleansing; fraenal ulceration; recession of the lingual gingiva. Ankyloglossia very rarely contributes to speech impairment.
(c) Usually none; lingual fraenectomy may be considered in severe cases.

23 (a) An inter-radicular abscess.
(b) Pulp therapy, or extract under antibiotic cover if medically indicated.

24 (a) The size and distribution of the marks suggest an adult bite.
(b) Further appointment to review dental situation. Activate local mechanisms for investigating non-accidental injuries.

25 (a) Observation. Removal may jeopardise the vitality of adjacent teeth. Surgery may be needed later if abnormalities develop.
(b) Cyst formation; resorption of the roots of the maxillary central incisors; ectopic eruption.

26 (a) Marked attrition.
(b) Bruxism and/or defective tooth formation.
(c) Bite plane to restore interocclusal height; composite restorations or crowns.

27 (a) Balloon on a string.
(b) Dentinogenesis imperfecta.

28 (a) Inflammation with smooth shiny areas and overgrowth of papillae.
(b) Anaemia or vitamin deficiency, particularly vitamin C.
(c) Blood screening, a haematological cause is the most likely.

29 (a) Leukaemia.
(b) Urgent haematology.
(c) Only palliative dental treatment to be undertaken until leukaemic remission is achieved. Extractions produce excessive haemorrhage.

30 (a) Bohn's nodules.
(b) Cystic degeneration of remnants of the dental lamina.
(c) Reassurance only, as the nodules will be shed spontaneously.

31 (a) Haemorrhage following damage to a blood vessel during injection.
(b) Cold compress to minimise swelling; reassurance; systemic antibiotics to prevent infection of the haematoma.

32 (a) Invagination.
(b) Infection and necrosis of the pulp with periapical involvement.
(c) By occluding palatal defect with fissure sealant or a restoration.

33 (a) A burn caused by beechwood creosote.
(b) Healing will be complete.
(c) In view of possible medico-legal action, full clinical notes are essential, if possible supported by diagrams or photographs.

34 (a) Natal teeth (mobile type).
(b) Extraction, as there is a danger of inhalation.
(c) Missing mandibular central incisors.

35 Consider non-accidental injury and activate local procedures; admit to hospital if concern is serious.

36 (a) Peripheral giant cell granuloma.
(b) Collagenous septa; giant cells; osteoid tissue.
(c) Excision, and curettage of underlying bone; there is a marked tendency for recurrence.

37 (a) Hypocalcification of mandibular first permanent molar; pericoronitis.
(b) Systemic upset in early infancy; occlusal trauma to a persistent operculum.
(c) Symptomatic relief of pericoronitis. The hypocalcification cannot be assessed until the tooth has erupted further.

38 (a) Dilaceration.
(b) Intrusion of the overlying primary incisor.
(c) Around 5 years, when root formation was beginning.

39 (a) Vital pulpotomy of mandibular first primary molar, missing second premolar.
(b) 5 years; the first permanent molar is very close to eruption since there is no overlying bone.
(c) Radiographic screening for other dental anomalies.

40 (a) Tuberculate supernumerary teeth palatal to the unerupted central incisors.
(b) Upper standard occlusal and periapical radiographs.
(c) Remove the supernumerary teeth and the retained primary incisors; maintain space; observe eruption of the permanent central incisors and expose if necessary.

41 (a) Tetracycline administration during tooth formation.
(b) The type, quantity and duration of tetracycline therapy.
(c) Bleaching; composite resin or porcelain veneers; possibly crowns later.

42 (a) Failure of the mandibular right first permanent molar to erupt; the contralateral tooth is fully erupted.
(b) Complex odontome; mandibular right second permanent molar absent.
(c) Remove odontome, review eruption of first permanent molar.

43 (a) Fronds of fibrous tissue covered by stratified squamous epithelium.
(b) Papilloma.

44 (a) A persistent labial fraenum has maintained a midline diastema.
(b) Fraenectomy and orthodontic treatment to approximate incisors and create good buccal occlusion.

45 (a) Frequent low pH carbonated drinks.
(b) Reduced calcium and phosphorus levels lower buffering power.

46 (a) Recurrent herpes labialis.
(b) Herpetic whitlow; herpetic ocular infection.
(c) Acyclovir cream.

47 (a) Dens in dente; invaginated odontome.
(b) Extraction. Consider the need to balance the extraction in order to minimise centre-line shift. It is possible that the contralateral tooth may be malformed.

48 (a) Papilloma.
(b) Excision biopsy.

49 (a) Dentinogenesis imperfecta.
(b) Autosomal dominant inheritance.

50 (a) Midline post-alveolar cleft; encephalocoele.
(b) Repair of cleft palate; neurosurgical repair of neural defect.

51 (a) Habitual scratching of the gum.
(b) Gingivitis artefacta.
(c) Treat local irritation; counsel the child and parents. Psychiatric help may be required in severe cases.

52 (a) Green stain.
(b) The action of chromogenic bacteria in established plaque.
(c) Mamellons.

53 (a) Asymmetrical open bite.
(b) Digit sucking.

54 (a) Surface zone (1), body of lesion (2), dark zone (3), translucent zone (4).
(b) Zones (1) and (3) are areas of reprecipitation, zones (2) and (4) are decalcification.

55 (a) The child has bitten the anaesthetised lip.
(b) Cold compress to minimise swelling; systemic antibiotics to prevent secondary infection.
(c) Inform parents; warn child; write careful notes.

56 (a) Extract the displaced teeth.
(b) Hypoplastic defects and/or dilaceration of the underlying permanent teeth. Attempts to reposition the displaced primary teeth would increase the likelihood of damage to the successors.

57 (a) Mucocoele (mucous retention cyst).
(b) Blockage of the duct in a minor salivary gland.
(c) Excision or marsupialization. There may be recurrence.

58 (a) Serial extraction.
(b) Extract all four primary canines, then the primary first molars, and then the first premolars.
(c) All unerupted teeth normal; Class I occlusion; mild crowding.

59 (a) Candidal infection under a removable orthodontic appliance.
(b) Improve hygiene of mouth and appliance; check fitting surface for roughness; if condition does not resolve, prescribe an antifungal drug eg miconazole gel.

60 (a) Bilateral cleft of lip and palate.
(b) Feeding, aesthetics.
(c) Counsel parents; fit feeding plate; use teat with large hole; early lip repair, with or without presurgical orthopaedic correction.

61 (a) Condylar fractures.
(b) Symptomatic relief; soft diet; exercise to encourage mobility and prevent ankylosis.

62 (a) Fusion of a mandibular primary central and lateral incisor.
(b) Fusion of two tooth germs.
(c) Absence of a permanent incisor.

63 (a) Inadequate trimming of bite plane during overjet reduction.
(b) Remove bite plane and continue retention.

64 (a) Cleidocranial dysplasia (Cleidocranial dysostosis).
(b) Partial or complete absence of clavicles.
(c) Frontal and parietal bossing; depressed nasal bridge; maxillary hypoplasia.
(d) Supernumerary teeth, associated with multiple unerupted teeth.

65 (a) Caries inside root canal; immature root apex; apical infection.
(b) Remove caries; endodontic treatment with intermediate calcium hydroxide dressing.
(c) Composite restoration incorporating labial veneer, post crown later.

66 (a) Hydrocephalus.
(b) Spina bifida.

67 (a) Accessory cusp; supernumerary premolar.
(b) Radiographs at different angulations.
(c) Continuity of tooth structure.

68 (a) Conical teeth; delayed exfoliation of primary teeth; hypodontia; midline diastema.
(b) Modify tooth shape using composite resin or crowns; orthodontics prior to prosthetics.
(c) Ectodermal dysplasia.

69 (a) Immature apices and periapical radiolucency.
(b) Orthograde root canal therapy using calcium hydroxide as an intermediate dressing to induce apical closure.

70 (a) An amalgam tattoo.
(b) Incorporation of amalgam particles in a primary tooth extraction socket.
(c) None, but reassure the parent that the appearance is not significant.

71 (a) Pulp death has produced an apical abscess and sinus associated with the right central incisor.
(b) Endodontics, with a calcium hydroxide dressing to induce an apical barrier.

72 (a) Giant cells; cellular fibrous tissue; many blood vessels; woven bone.
(b) Giant cell lesion.

73 (a) Epidemic parotitis (Mumps).
(b) Inflammation of the papilla at the opening to the parotid duct.

74 (a) Submergence.
(b) Ankylosis.
(c) Extraction if submergence becomes severe. Consider a space maintainer.

75 Missing maxillary left lateral incisor; centre lines not coincident; peg right lateral incisor.

76 Epidermolysis bullosa (simplex and dystrophic types); pemphigus; bullous erythema multiforme. In this case the diagnosis was epidermolysis bullosa dystrophica.

77 (a) Congenital porphyria.
(b) Defective breakdown of haemoglobin molecules.

78 (a) An angioneurotic reaction has produced multiple petechial haemorrhages.
(b) Haematology; test for sensitivity to local anaesthetic.

79 Papillon-Lefèvre syndrome; Histiocytosis-X; leukaemia; neutropenia; acrodynia; hypophosphatasia; acatalasia; Chediak-Higashi syndrome; prepubertal periodontitis. In this case the diagnosis was Papillon-Lefèvre syndrome.

80 (a) Amelogenesis imperfecta (hypoplastic type).
(b) A genetic defect which affects ameloblast function.

81 (a) Crouzon's syndrome (craniofacial dysostosis).
(b) Naso-maxillary hypoplasia; exorbitism; divergent squint; flat forehead.
(c) Severe class III malocclusion with open bite.

82 (a) Gross calculus; gingival inflammation; calcification defects.
(b) Scaling; oral hygiene instruction; restoration of the first premolars.
(c) Assisted oral hygiene measures.

83 (a) Talon cusp.
(b) Appearance; occlusal interference.
(c) Progressive reduction and desensitisation; endodontics may be required.

84 (a) A band and loop space maintainer.
(b) Premature loss of a second primary molar from an intact dentition.

85 (a) Dentinogenesis imperfecta; hereditary opalescent dentine.
(b) Attrition; periapical infection; poor appearance.

86 (a) Facial asymmetry; absent pinna.
(b) Oculoauriculovertebral dysplasias.
(c) First branchial arch syndrome.

87, 88 (a) Dentigerous cyst on unerupted permanent maxillary lateral incisor.
(b) Displacement of teeth; destruction of bone; infection.
(c) Extract retained primary lateral incisor and canine; marsupialize cyst.

89 (a) Dehiscence of labial bone.
(b) Labial displacement of the associated tooth.
(c) Very careful oral hygiene. Surgery is not beneficial.

90 (a) Sublingual dermoid cyst.
(b) Bimanual palpation; transillumination; aspiration.
(c) Surgical removal.

91 (a) Submerging primary molars; delayed eruption of permanent teeth; lack of enamel.
(b) Deficiency of somatotrophic hormone or thyroxine may have affected tooth eruption. The enamel deficiency is hereditary amelogenesis imperfecta of the hypoplastic type.

92 (a) Unilateral facial paralysis.
(b) Idiopathic (Bell's palsy); cranial neuropathy; herpes; sarcoidosis.

93 (a) Eruption cyst.
(b) Reassurance; hard teething toys. Resolution is usually spontaneous and surgical intervention is rarely necessary.

94 (a) Submergence of first and second primary molars; impaction of first permanent molar.
(b) High tooth-tissue ratio; ankylosis of primary molars; ectopic eruption of first permanent molar.
(c) Retain submerged teeth as space maintainers, extract if submergence becomes severe and consider a space maintaining appliance. Attempt to disimpact the first permanent molar.

95 (a) Cotton wool 'burn' caused by removal of a dry cotton wool roll.
(b) Moisten cotton wool roll before removal.

96 (a) Calculus in the right submandibular duct (Wharton's duct).
(b) Pain and swelling of the submandibular salivary gland at mealtimes.
(c) Bimanual palpation to milk stone from duct; if unsuccessful remove surgically.
(d) Haematological and biochemical screening for alkaline phosphatase levels.

97 (a) Dentinogenesis imperfecta; tetracycline stain.
(b) Family history; medical history; attrition; distribution of discoloration.
(c) Radiographs would confirm dentinogenesis imperfecta. Yellow fluorescence with ultraviolet light would confirm tetracycline.

98 (a) Acute herpetic gingivostomatitis.
(b) By contact; often by over-enthusiastic kissing of the child by an adult carrier.
(c) High fluid intake; soft food; systemic antibiotics for secondary infection.

99 (a) Hypodontia; small teeth; sparse eyebrows; fine hair; frontal bossing; depressed nose; prominent ears.
(b) Ectodermal dysplasia.
(c) Hypohidrotic form is X-linked recessive. Autosomal dominant and recessive forms also occur.

100 (a) A Turner tooth.
(b) Involvement of the follicle of the developing premolar by infection from a primary predecessor.

101 (a) Retention of mucus.
(b) A mucocoele (mucous retention cyst).
(c) In association with a major or minor salivary gland.

102 (a) Tetracycline administration during tooth formation.
(b) Incorporation of drug into the mineral matrix produces a chromogenic structure.
(c) A wide band of discoloration.

103 (a) Scleroderma.
(b) Localised areas of periodontal destruction, followed by tooth ankylosis.
(c) Sharpey's fibres are replaced by disorganised collagen with focal hyalinisation.

104 (a) Treacher-Collins syndrome (mandibulofacial dysostosis).
(b) Dysplastic ears; hypoplasia of zygoma; hypoplasia of body of mandible.
(c) Pharyngeal hypoplasia may lead to difficulty with intubation.

105 (a) Discoloured banding; the enamel hypoplasia is related to systemic disturbance.
(b) Cystic fibrosis. Alternative antibiotics are now used; recent improvements in management have meant that not all sufferers require maintenance on long-term antibiotic prophylaxis.

106 (a) A conical supernumerary tooth (mesiodens).
(b) Supplemental lateral incisor; tuberculate supernumerary; odontome.

107 (a) Transposition of the mandibular lateral incisor.
(b) Ectopic eruption following abnormal crypt position.

108 (a) Trauma from the coil of a Roberts retractor.
(b) Fit a new appliance with an alternative incisor retractor. The ulcer will heal spontaneously.

109 (a) Careful débridement to prevent tattooing.
(b) Check adequacy of tetanus protection; consider systemic antibiotics.

110 (a) Aphthous ulcer.
(b) Recurrent ulcers of this severity indicate the need for haematology and possibly jejunal biopsy.
(c) Anaemia; Crohn's disease; coeliac disease.

111, 112 (a) Oro-facial granulomatosis.
(b) Patch test for food allergy; jejunal biopsy.
(c) Dietary avoidance advice; steroid therapy.

113 (a) Premature resorption and bone loss involving second primary molars; drift of mandibular incisors.
(b) Biopsy; haematology; immunology.
(c) Prepubertal periodontitis associated with Histiocytosis-X.

114 (a) Rh positive foetus in a previously sensitised Rh negative mother.
(b) Erythroblastosis foetalis (Rhesus incompatibility).
(c) Enamel formed *in utero* is defective. Postnatal enamel is normal, producing a rhesus hump.

115 (a) Scleroderma.
(b) Diffuse fibrosis of skin and other tissues, including the periodontium.
(c) Unknown, there appears to be an immunological basis.

116 (a) Bulbosity; irregular dentinal tubules; reduced scalloping of amelo-dentinal junction; pulpal obliteration.
(b) Dentinogenesis imperfecta.

117 (a) About six months.
(b) Coeliac disease, produced by allergy to gluten.
(c) All first permanent molars, the permanent maxillary central incisors and canines.

118 (a) Gross caries affecting maxillary teeth; a sinus above the right canine.
(b) Extract unsaveable teeth; consider a denture.
(c) Restrict the frequency of sugar intake.

119 Submucous cleft of palate; defective velopharyngeal seal, causing speech problems.

120 (a) 7-8 years.
(b) Low tooth-tissue ratio; abnormal fraenum; incisive canal cyst; midline supernumerary tooth; a missing lateral incisor.

121 (a) Osteogenesis imperfecta (tarda type).
(b) Mesodermal deficiency produces thin sclera allowing the choroid to show through.
(c) Dentinogenesis imperfecta.

122 (a) Oral iron therapy.
(b) Swallow tablets or capsules whole; suck elixir through a straw.

123 (a) By intrusion of the left primary central incisor during calcification of the permanent successor.
(b) About one year old. Approximately one quarter of the crown was calcified when the trauma occurred.
(c) Remove tip and prepare for composite restoration; endodontics and post crown may be necessary.

124 (a) Trauma; pulp death; haemosiderin in dentinal tubules.
(b) Endodontics, followed by bleaching; composite or porcelain veneer, or post crown.

125 (a) Papillon-Lefèvre syndrome (hyperkeratosis palmoplantaris and periodontoclasia).
(b) Plaque control and root planing; extract unsaveable teeth; long-term antibiotics.

126 (a) Down's syndrome.
(b) Mid-face hypoplasia; small nose with flattened bridge; mongoloid slant to eyes; Brushfield spots on iris; broad fissured lips.
(c) Abnormality of chromosome 21 with trisomy or translocation.

127 (a) Fissuring and papillary hypertrophy.
(b) Down's syndrome.
(c) Stagnation and debris in fissures may lead to infection.
(d) Good oral hygiene and active tongue cleansing. Surgical tongue reduction may be considered.

128 (a) Gemination of the maxillary left central incisor to produce a double tooth.
(b) By partial dichotomy of one tooth germ.
(c) Poor morphology of the tooth indicates a need for extraction followed by an etch retained bridge.

129 (a) Anterior open bite and unilateral cross bite.
(b) Prolonged dummy sucking.
(c) The open bite will probably improve following cessation of the habit. Cross bite is liable to persist.

130 (a) A lymphoma that produces lymph node enlargement.
(b) Sternberg-Reed giant cells.
(c) Dental development has been arrested by irradiation of cervical lymph nodes.

131 (a) Tooth/tissue ratio; age of patient; type of teeth lost.
(b) The primary teeth.
(c) The leeway space.

132 (a) 50 mg of sodium fluoride per 1 ml of varnish.
(b) 22.1 mg per ml.

133 (a) High fluoride intake during tooth formation.
(b) Accentuated perikymata; striae; symmetry about midline.

134 (a) Ulceration beneath tongue when suckling.
(b) Smooth incisal edges or extract.

135 (a) Missing second premolar; submerged second primary molar; impacted third permanent molar.
(b) Extract submerged tooth, partial or complete space closure using a fixed appliance.
(c) Poor prognosis of submerged tooth; impaction of third molar.

136 (a) Tetracycline administration during tooth formation.
(b) During the 3rd trimester of pregnancy.
(c) Ultraviolet fluorescence; medical history of mother.

137 (a) Developing unilateral facial hyperplasia.
(b) Radiographs; blood biochemistry, including alkaline phosphatase levels; biopsy.
(c) Fibrous dysplasia.

138 (a) Dilaceration of the crown of the lateral incisor.
(b) Between 18 months and 2 years of age.
(c) Intrusion of primary lateral incisor on to the more palatally placed follicle of the permanent tooth.

139 (a) A midline conical supernumerary tooth (mesiodens).
(b) Conical pointed crown and long, fine root.
(c) Over 50 per cent occur in the premaxilla.

140 (a) Maintain oral cleanliness; check tetanus protection; systemic antibiotics.
(b) Await re-eruption but orthodontic extrusion and realignment are likely to be needed.

141 (a) Impetigo.
(b) Coagulase positive staphylococci.
(c) Direct contact; infected fomites; poor hygiene.

142 (a) Radiographs; electric pulp tests.
(b) Protect exposed dentine and restore crown shape.

143 (a) Cyanosis.
(b) Cyanotic heart disease—most probably Fallot's tetralogy.
(c) Avoid general anaesthesia; give prophylactic antibiotics for any procedure that may cause bleeding.

144 (a) Extensive bone loss distal to the central incisors; widened periodontal ligament space left central incisor.
(b) Iatrogenic, due to excessive force and apical migration by an elastic band.

145 Class III malocclusion; hypodontia; periodontal disease.

146 (a) Asymmetry; flat forehead; hypertelorism; exorbitism; strabismus; underdeveloped maxilla.
(b) Crouzon's syndrome (craniofacial dysostosis).
(c) Crowding in upper arch; anterior open bite; class III malocclusion; high arched palate.

147 (a) Radiographs to check for root fracture and a pellet in the soft tissues; pulp vitality tests.
(b) Removable splint for 1-3 weeks.

148 (a) Epidermolysis bullosa dystrophica.
(b) Severe oral ulceration, often produced by toothbrushing or dental treatment.
(c) Probably a mesodermal defect affecting collagen metabolism.

149 (a) Fleshy fraenum; midline diastema; supplemental mandibular incisor.
(b) None at present. The diastema may close when the permanent canines erupt and the mandibular arch is well aligned.

150 (a) Amelogenesis imperfecta (hypoplastic type with random pitting and grooving).
(b) The 'Lyon hypothesis'. Females have vertical banding, males have thin enamel.
(c) Aesthetics and hypersensitivity.

151 (a) Endogenous tongue thrust.
(b) Lisp; high gonial angle; proclined mandibular incisors.

152 (a) Drug induced (phenytoin) gingival fibromatosis.
(b) Meticulous plaque control; gingivectomy.
(c) Continued meticulous plaque control. Consult physician concerning a change of medication.

153 (a) Occipitomental view.
(b) A fluid level in the right maxillary antrum suggestive of sinusitis.
(c) Antibiotics and decongestants.

154 (a) Pierre-Robin syndrome.
(b) Maintain airway.
(c) Good, the retrognathism improves with age.

155 (a) Arrested caries.
(b) High and frequent sugar intake in the past.
(c) Retention of the teeth as space maintainers.

156 (a) A skin graft.
(b) Sulcus deepening procedure: this treatment is now obsolete, since long-term results were unsatisfactory.

157 (a) Hand, foot and mouth disease.
(b) Reassurance and symptomatic relief is adequate for most affected children. Immunocompromised patients require antiviral therapy eg acyclovir.

158 (a) Chronological hypoplasia (incremental hypoplasia).
(b) Systemic disturbance during the second year of life.

159 (a) Enamel hypoplasia and root dilaceration.
(b) Trauma to the primary central incisor during maturation of the enamel of the permanent tooth.

160 (a) Congenital epulis; granular cell myoblastoma.
(b) Excision biopsy.
(c) Good, recurrence is unlikely following total excision.

161 (a) Pulpotomy (partial pulpectomy).
(b) Induction of apical closure using calcium hydroxide after canal preparation.
(c) Steroid-containing endodontic preparations; paraformaldehyde preparations.

162 (a) Enamel erosion.
(b) Dietary indiscretion; frequent drinks of lemon juice.
(c) Composite resin restorations; diet advice.

163 (a) Displacement of the first permanent molar.
(b) Excision biopsy.
(c) Fibro-epithelial polyp; giant cell lesion (biopsy confirmed this).

164 (a) Cyanosis; finger clubbing.
(b) Pulmonary stenosis; ventricular septal defect; an over-riding aorta; compensatory right ventricular hypertrophy.

165 (a) Anterior fontanelle.
(b) 1-2 years.

166 (a) 'Ugly duckling stage'.
(b) Pressure from unerupted permanent canines on the roots of the lateral incisors. Eruption of the canines tends to move the incisor crowns together.

167 (a) Etched enamel prisms.
(b) Orthophosphoric acid of 30-50 per cent concentration.

168 (a) Apert's syndrome (acrocephalosyndactyly type I).
(b) Flat forehead; naso-maxillary hypoplasia; syndactyly.

169 (a) Mandibular right primary canine, lateral and central incisors, the left central and lateral incisors are fused. The left primary canine is normal.
(b) Increased incidence of hypodontia, especially lower incisors.

170 (a) There is more than one cause. Mesiodens just visible; missing right primary lateral incisor; one or both permanent lateral incisors possibly missing; fleshy fraenum; racial characteristic.
(b) None—await further eruption of mesiodens, then extract.

171 (a) A Spitz-Holter valve.
(b) Hydrocephaly.
(c) The ventricles of the brain and the subclavian vein or mediastinum.

172 (a) Extraction.
(b) Space loss; centre line shift.

173 (a) A band of hypoplasia and hypocalcification.
(b) Measles.
(c) 8-10 months: the central incisors are the most affected.

174 (a) Extensive erosion palatally on the primary incisors. Abscess on left primary central incisor.
(b) Low pH drinks in a bottle or reservoir feeder.

175 (a) Chronic trauma due to parafunctional activity, such as nocturnal bruxism.
(b) Advice; an occlusal guard may be necessary.

176 (a) Vesicles.
(b) Hand, foot and mouth disease.
(c) Coxsackie virus, usually type A-16.

177 (a) Chlorhexidine digluconate mouth-rinse.
(b) Adsorption of chlorhexidine on to hydroxyapatite.
(c) By the use of conventional toothpaste before the mouth-rinse.

178 (a) Pink spot.
(b) Internal resorption, possibly following trauma.
(c) Extraction.

179 (a) Expansion of the buccal alveolar plate; bluish swelling.
(b) Radiographs; excision biopsy.
(c) Central giant cell lesion.

180 (a) Apical root resorption.
(b) Poor.
(c) Keep the central incisors as space maintainers until mobility necessitates extraction.

181 (a) Pulp death; ankylosis; re-eruption failure.
(b) Delayed exfoliation; hypoplasia or dilaceration of the permanent successor.

182 (a) It is associated with teething.
(b) Local—teething toys or teething foods; apply teething gel to gums. Systemic—analgesics and hypnotics if needed.

183 (a) Missing maxillary lateral incisors; enamel mottling;notch left central incisor; extrinsic stain.
(b) Heredity; localised ameloblast damage; attrition; chromogenic bacteria.

184 (a) 7-8 years.
(b) Acute herpetic gingivostomatitis.
(c) Encourage fluid intake; advise soft bland diet; systemic antibiotics for secondary infection.

185 (a) Perlèche.
(b) Lip licking habit.
(c) Cessation of habit; application of barrier cream.

186 (a) A cavernous haemangioma of lip and tongue.
(b) Good; hamartomas grow with the child and may regress when somatic growth ceases.
(c) Avoid extractions by a strict preventive regime.

187 (a) Hemifacial atrophy (Romberg's syndrome).
(b) Facial asymmetry due to unilateral atrophy of bone and muscle.
(c) Contralateral Jacksonian epilepsy; trigeminal neuralgia.

188 (a) A large fleshy labial fraenum.
(b) Oral hygiene instruction. Surgery is avoided in the primary dentition since the fraenum may regress.

189 (a) Repaired cleft palate with scarring and fistula; candidal infection of mucosa.
(b) Improved hygiene of mouth and obturator; check fitting surface of obturator; antifungal drugs.

190 (a) Either gemination of the central incisors or fusion of the right central and lateral incisors and of the left central incisor with a supernumerary tooth to give double teeth.
(b) Pulp morphology; dental crowding; occlusion; appearance.

191 Two retained maxillary primary incisors; an odontome preventing eruption of the maxillary left permanent incisors.

192 (a) Phenytoin hyperplasia.
(b) The phenytoin produces exaggerated growth of fibroblasts and epithelium in response to gingival irritation.
(c) Prophylaxis followed by meticulous plaque control may induce regression.

193 (a) Gingivitis artefacta.
(b) Habitual picking of the gum with a finger-nail.
(c) Gingival recession, producing a long clinical crown.

194 (a) Ranula.
(b) Sublingual dermoid cyst; Ludwig's angina.
(c) No fever; bimanual palpation; transillumination; aspiration.
(d) In the body or duct of the sublingual salivary gland.

195 (a) Lesch-Nyhan syndrome.
(b) A disorder of purine metabolism.
(c) Arm splints; dental extractions for severe cases.

196 (a) Dental abscess; boil; actinomycosis.
(b) Eliminate dental causes; prescribe systemic antibiotics; if there is no resolution, test for actinomycosis.

197 (a) Bulbous crowns; cervical constrictions; short roots; calcified pulps; periapical areas.
(b) Dentinogenesis imperfecta.

198 (a) Dietary indiscretions, including frequent carbonated beverages.
(b) Dietary analysis.
(c) Modify diet; apply topical fluoride; restore with composite resin or veneers.

199 (a) Frontal plagiocephaly.
(b) Premature fusion of one right or left coronal suture.
(c) Tilted occlusal plane; dental arch asymmetry.

200 (a) Arrested caries; palatally displaced second premolar.
(b) Aggressive caries in the primary and early mixed dentition.
(c) Extract first permanent molar and align second premolar.

201 (a) Fracture of maxillary central incisor with widened periodontal ligament space; supernumerary tooth; resorbed apex lateral incisor.
(b) Endodontics to left central and lateral incisors followed by extraction of the supernumerary tooth.

Index

Numbers refer to illustrations